INJURY FREE

MENTAL TRAINING FOR ELITE ATHLETES

BY RICHARD MALONEY

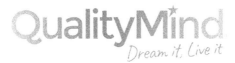

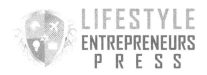

Copyright © 2019 Richard Maloney

All rights reserved. No part of this book may be reproduced or transmitted in any form or by any means, electronic or mechanical, including photocopying, recording, or by an information storage and retrieval system — except by a reviewer who may quote brief passages in a review to be printed in a magazine or newspaper — without permission in writing from the publisher.

ISBN 978-1950367238

Table of Contents

Foreword by Shaun Higgins 6
Prelude by Richard Maloney 9
The Quality Mind Model 15
   Now Download the Quality Mind App 17
Introduction 20
   What is the Real Cost of Injuries in Professional Sport? 21
   The 5 Key Areas Where Athletes Break Down 23
Ben Jacobs: Case Study 28
Intelligent Energy Management 34
The Five Steps To Creating a Quality Mind 42
Step #1: Evaluate 45
   Activity #1: Life Scorecard Assessment 46
   What Do You Seriously Want? 50
   Bottom line: If You Can't See It, You Can't Create It 51
Case Study: Shaun Higgins 53
Step #2: Retrain 59
   The Journey of Three Stages 59
   We're Always Creating Anyway 61
   Vehicle / Explorer / Intuition 64
   The Four A's 67
   Practice Makes Perfect 74
   Delving into Thought Shopping 76
   Activity #2: Dreams and Fears 80
   The Six Stages of Mindful Alignment 82
   Four Universal Laws for Mindfulness 85
   How Are You Vibing? 88
   Activity #3: Designing the New You (Part 1) 92
   Activity #4: Meditation – 10-Day Beginners Series 95
Case Study: Tiarna Ernst 96
Step #3: Clean 103

    Limiting Beliefs. 106
    The Four Stages of Diffusing Old Beliefs 108
    Activity #5: Remove Limiting Beliefs Meditation. 109
    What You Think is What You Get. 110
    Your Mirror Reflection. 112
    Inner World VS Outer World 116
    Why is Understanding Our DNA Important?. 117
    Activity #6: How Do I Recode Myself?. 118
    Love & Forgiveness 119
    Activity #7: Questions to Reveal the Gifts of Your Reflection
    to Love & Forgive. 120
Case Study: Easton Wood 121
Step #4: Dream 124
    Discovering Synchronicity 124
    Recognizing Contrast 125
    Abundance 127
    See It, Feel It, Become It. Close the Gap 128
    Activity #8: Designing the New You (Part 2 of Activity 3). 129
Case Study: Trent Dumont 131
Case Study: Laura Attard 136
Step #5: Live. 141
    QM Performance Plan. 141
    To Truly Live – Live With Heart. 143
    7 Non Negotiables. 145
Backmatter 148
    Acknowledgments. 148
    About the Author. 150
    Further Information 152

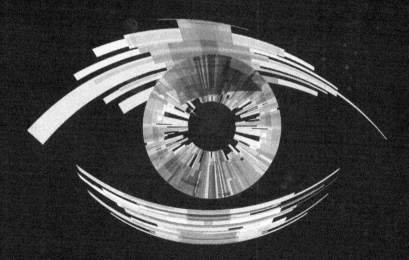

Foreword
by Shaun Higgins

I have been involved with Richard Maloney and the Quality Mind Program in some capacity since 2011. We first met when I was playing for the Western Bulldogs Football Club in the Australian Football League (AFL) and Richard joined the club as our Leadership & Culture Coach. His teachings were unique and exciting, and he offered a fresh and convincing approach that none of us had ever encountered before. His program really resonated with me, and I enjoyed the knowledge. It all made perfect sense, however, at the time I was very young, and for whatever reason, I wasn't really applying what I was learning consistently. Our working relationship at the club strengthened over the years, and Richard began to offer me one on one guidance as part of the program. What I was learning from him was both powerful and compelling, but still something was holding me back from really taking the leap and doing the daily inner work I knew I needed to do in order to flourish in football and in life. I continued to dabble in Richard's teachings, and I continued to idle in my football career.

The turning point for me was undoubtedly my injury in 2013. After round two of the 2013 AFL season, I was walking past Richard in the corridor on the Monday morning when he pulled me aside to talk. I'll never forget his words on that day. He said "we need to catch up Hig. It looks like you've got a few pressures going on and I can see that we *need* to have a chat." We made a plan to get together the following week, and then he said "be careful this weekend."

That Sunday, just 6 days after our conversation in the corridor, I broke my foot so severely that I was sidelined for the next 12 months and my football career was on the brink of being over. When I look back on the lead up to that fateful day, all I can remember is how I felt before that life changing round three game. I was sitting at home on the floor trying to prepare myself mentally, and all I could think about was the pressure of it all. Extreme heaviness, burden, low energy, fear and dread. Quite simply, I didn't want to play.

At that point in my career I was seen by most as an unfulfilled talent that had the skills and the ability to be the best, but who never consistently played at the level he should be playing at. I was constantly riddled with injury, so I was only ever achieving sporadic success. And now here I was at rock bottom, staring at the bleak possibility of having to start over doing something else with my life entirely. It was an ominous prospect, and Richard's words haunted me.

I had surgery on my foot and I had 12 months to really go to work on myself, which I did with Richard's guidance. He challenged me not to come back to football at all unless I was ready to change myself from the inside out and be the best version of myself — not only as a player, but also as a man. That year of self-discovery broadened my horizons on every level, and I realized that my status quo wasn't good enough for me anymore. I had always known where I wanted to go in life, and who I wanted to be, I just didn't know how to get there, and I always felt a separation between who I was and who I wanted to be, both on and off the field. Upon reflection, I knew that there was always a noticeable correlation between how I was feeling in terms of my energy levels, thoughts and feelings, and my overall performance; however, I was not at all aware of this at the time.

After successfully returning to the game in 2014, I had become that better version of myself, and I ultimately made the decision to leave the Western Bulldogs FC — the club I never thought I'd leave. Before working with Richard and living the Quality Mind program daily, I never would have had the courage to take that leap by choice. It was a major turning point for me, and I continued to engage Richard's services as he frequently challenged me to let go of my limiting beliefs. He challenged me to be best and fairest — which led to two club best and fairest awards, then he challenged me to be All Australian (AFL) — which I achieved. To this day, he is still successfully challenging me to let go consistently of what's holding me back.

The QM program, for me, represents continual growth, and I'm forever learning, evolving and manifesting more for myself. I still slip back into my old mental programming, but now when that happens I'm aware of it and I'm fully aware of what the repercussions will be if I don't turn my thinking around. In the past, I wouldn't have had a clue how to do that, but now I just turn to the Quality Mind app, follow the steps, and

I'm back in my optimum head-space, forgetting the 'how' and the 'when' and just focussing on the 'NOW'.

Like so many of us, my temperament means I'm always wanting to control the situation or the outcome. This doesn't serve me well — and without intervention, that would have always been my default mode. The QM program gives you a clear vision and a control mechanism. If you can't see it for yourself, you can't create it, and therefore you can't live it. You have to want it first and foremost, but even when you have a clear vision of what you want, you need to let go of the limiting beliefs that will hold you back from getting to where you want to go.

Today, I am the footballer I always knew I was capable of being, and I also feel I have plenty more to offer at the age of 32, when most players are retiring or being delisted. I've just signed with North Melbourne FC for two more years, and my future has never felt brighter. The Quality Mind app has become a crucial part of my daily life, and it continually reminds me to check in with myself, make sure I'm in the NOW, make sure I continue to keep my excitement levels up and make sure I'm vibrating on a really high energy.

In closing, I can confidently say that the Quality Mind program categorically saved my football career. It transformed my life and got me back on track, enabling me to achieve the clarity and mental strength required to first identify my dreams and then to fulfil them. Now I dream it and I live it every day.

Enjoy the journey!

Prelude
by Richard Maloney

From a very early age, I felt like I was here for a reason. I didn't know why, and I had no idea what I'd been delivered here to do, but I sensed that it would unfold and be revealed to me someday, and so I waited. In the mean-time, I didn't take life or people too seriously, and often this seemingly relaxed approach worked to my detriment. At school, I was completely disengaged with the curriculum, the teachers, and their teaching methods, and this resulted in me being perceived as a difficult, combative, problem child.

As the years passed and my disenchantment for the status quo intensified, the perception that I was more trouble than I was worth also heightened, and I was ultimately asked to leave two different schools. I struggled to fit into the 'box' that my parents and teachers expected me to fit into, and so it was assumed that I was non-academic and wholly incapable of applying myself. I found this frustrating because I knew this wasn't who I really was, but I also felt misunderstood, and at times just completely defeated. If they couldn't see me for me, then what was the point?

Sport, however, was my one saving grace. It offered me a platform to excel and exhibit my talents, an outlet for my frustrations, and an opportunity to mould myself into society through my passion. I was not only accepted, but also continually recognized and rewarded for my talents, and it felt like the one place where conforming was an option. Unfortunately though, this one safe haven in my life was still not enough for me to overcome my other demons, and I really struggled mentally throughout my teens. I felt discouraged, misunderstood and pigeon holed as "the bad guy," and at the age of 16, I even considered taking my own life. At this point I still had no clear sense of purpose, and no real sense of self. I knew I wasn't who people thought I was, but if I wasn't that, then who was I?

During this tumultuous period, my sporting abilities continued to flourish and I was recruited to the St Kilda Football Club in the Australian Football League. This was the epitome of success for a footballer, and on the surface, it seemed like a dream come true. The opportunity to play football at the most elite level in Australia — and as one of the Saints, the team I had idolised my entire life! Everyone thought I was living the dream, and yet, what I gained there was a very stark and unnerving realization that my attitude towards people, competition, and life in general was rather ruthless and unhealthy—and I didn't even possess the distinction of being the best anymore. I'd gone from being the biggest fish in a small pond to a small fish in an ocean.

Other elite footballers were just as good as I was, if not better, and even more importantly, they also had the right mindset. I struggled with the pressure of performing to a higher standard, and with the ego hit that came with no longer being the standout player. I had always been one of the best in class, and this had come easily. Now, I had to work so hard and continually strive to prove myself to my peers and coaches. I felt discouraged and disillusioned. My young ego copped consistent beatings, and ultimately, I got injured. From there, sadly, I just quit.

One of the other reasons I think I had such a bad attitude at the time was one of the all too familiar classics—my parents got divorced. It was far from amicable and the raw pain and inner turmoil this inflicted was profound, and lingering. My mum had a break-down of sorts, and my sister was overseas at the time so it all fell on me, and I felt an instinctive need to take care of her, along with an overwhelming sense of looming responsibility. A lot for any teenager, and just all too much for me.

At the same time, I also experienced the shock of almost losing my best mate Jason, who had been my closest friend (like a brother) from the age of 5. He and his mum were on a road trip when they were involved in a car accident on the West Gate Bridge in Melbourne. A collision at the top of the bridge sent the car into the safety rail, potentially causing a plummet of 58 meters (or 190 feet) into the Yarra River. This terrifying experience sent my best friend into a downward spiral of post-traumatic stress which brought on panic attacks and anxiety. Jase wasn't really the same after that.

Jase and I were still just kids, but we were both going through our own private hell, and we both felt like we were drowning as our old worlds seemingly dissolved around us. At the time, I was too lost and broken myself to help Jase in any meaningful way. But caring for my mother post-divorce, and stepping up as the man of the house forced me to mature swiftly, and I became obsessed with the concept of WHY? Why did one near death experience change my best friend so profoundly overnight, and why was I so quick to throw away my opportunity for greatness at the first sign of struggle?

Through our paralleled suffering, I unearthed my true passion for working to understand the human mind, to understand myself, and to help my best mate Jase. I became obsessed by the concepts of metaphysics, and I felt a deep need to explore and uncover just why we were here. I started by researching all of the major religions, then exploring the science of the mind and psychology. From there I ventured farther afield, with theories of parallel dimensions and the direction of personal energy. Along the way, I met many interesting kindred spirits who offered new perspectives and ideas that felt right — thoughts that I added to my ever-growing mental mosaic of life's meaning.

Over the course of these 'seeking' years, I was also playing football at the State League levels at numerous clubs throughout Australia. This is one level down from the AFL that so elusively escaped me, and where I was often the leader or captain, and the enforcer on the field. I thrived in physical combat because I found this allowed me to gain a major advantage over my competitor mentally. I had always pushed the boundaries of being overly physical with footy, and yet off the field, I could so often be found meditating and looking deeper into spirituality. I was quite the walking contradiction, and I was concerned about people knowing that I wore two such radically different hats. This insecurity began to intensify as I came to the realization that my life seemed to be contradictory on so many levels. Here I was, known for being the enforcer, yet I was also a young man on a mystical journey. Aggression and harmony were my two driving forces in life, and in my mind, the two didn't really connect as one person — which only exacerbated my uncertainty as to who I was, and why we were here.

In the years that followed, I thankfully matured both as an athlete and as a man, and I continued along a leadership path, both in sport and at work. I also began to uncover notable patterns in elite athletes and business clients, and this sparked a keen interest which prompted me to study psychology, life coaching, NLP and hypnotherapy, just to name a few. For the first time in my life, I had unearthed a deep passion for learning, and I couldn't get enough of it!

As my studies progressed and I continued to explore, I was surprised to learn that no one was offering a clear and tangible system with a step-by-step structure to take me (or anyone, for that matter) from A (lost, confused, prioritizing petty energies) to Z (self-aware, focused, passionate and on the fast track towards success). This was what I knew I needed and what I'd been searching for, and so while my search continued, the Quality Mind program unwittingly started to emerge in my mind.

I continued along my path as an employee working for others, both as an athlete, and as a coach in sport and business, all the while still learning, researching, building and adding to my mental mosaic for my own future business. Visualizing, testing and trialling how to most effectively return athletes and others to their early standards of high performance and beyond, by treating all areas that need to be in balance — the body, the mind and the soul.

My broad and varied experience over the years as an athlete, a contractor and an employee led me to experience incredible roles and learning curves with over 80 sports teams within some of Australia's best sporting associations. I was associated with 7 elite sporting clubs, which included St Kilda Football Club, Melbourne Football Club, Fremantle Football Club, Western Bulldogs Football Club, Melbourne Storm Rugby League, Melbourne Tigers Basketball and Melbourne Vixens Netball. I was also working with nonprofessional sporting teams, and I helped lead these teams to 45 grand finals for 35 winning championships.

The wealth of experience I gained here allowed me to recognise patterns in strong leadership, culture, and high performance. I also identified patterns in low-performing teams and businesses, and I set out to develop a step-by-step process that subliminally activated people to create rapid business success. This was the beginning of Engage & Grow Global, my globally-recognized program that reconnects and reinvigorates employees in the workplace. I sent it out to the world online and, within four years, we found ourselves in 80 countries with over 300 licensed coaches. Our carefully defined and systemized approach has resonated with thousands of now-engaged employees. We help to 'wake them up,' thus enabling them to realize their true potential. We have customized a unique 'Group Activation System' for every business, which addresses their specific needs and goals.

This experience and success put me on firm ground as I built the bedrock for Quality Mind, which I'd unknowingly been building via my 'mental mosaic' from the age of 19. I now understood that everyone creates and is responsible for their own reality, every minute of every day. This applies to all of us, including athletes, and when I applied this theory to athletes who get injured, surely it made sense to also assume that injuries must also be part of an athletes creation on some level?

More years passed, and as Engage & Grow Global exploded, I continued to build on my lifelong passion project — Quality Mind — with the understanding that one day soon, I would pass the Engage & Grow reigns on, allowing me to put all of my time and focus into my QM business. That time has now come, and I know without question that the body is led by the mind, and that you can't hide from yourself. Injuries, illness and disease can all reflect an area of challenge in your life, and patterned injuries taking place in the elite sports world are often caused by insecurities in your own head. Here's the thing, subconsciously and unconsciously, your body will make every effort to keep you safe by default, and it will shut down in certain stressful scenarios to protect you.

Nine times out of ten, I can now accurately predict when an athlete I'm working with is going to get injured, and through my twenty years of working with high-performing people and athletes, I've built a tangible, proven, step by step system to eradicate injury and improve performance.

I began trialling my system on athletes in 2015, and they experienced immediate and notable success and improvement. This resulted in a flurry of media coverage.

In 2015 I also trialled the program on my best mate Jase, who was still really struggling with his same anxious demons all these years on. I used a lot of trial and error on him, and as he gained traction and understood the process more, we were able to build something amazing together. A life-changing strategy that finally enabled him to turn a corner, and one he hasn't looked back from since. We created the universal 'Personal Activation System' — a system that works for everyday people, not just athletes.

Before I knew it, I had more Quality Mind business than I could handle. Meanwhile, Engage & Grow Global was really taking off across the world as well, enabling me to travel the globe for 4 months of each year. I

The following is just one example; a snippet from The Herald Sun Newspaper on December 12th, 2015. Written by Glenn McFarlane, (Picture: Jake Nowakowski) the article can be viewed in its entirety on our website. https://www.qualitymindglobal.com/blog/article/easton-wood-shaun-higgins-credit-injury-free-mind-coach-with-career-best-seasons

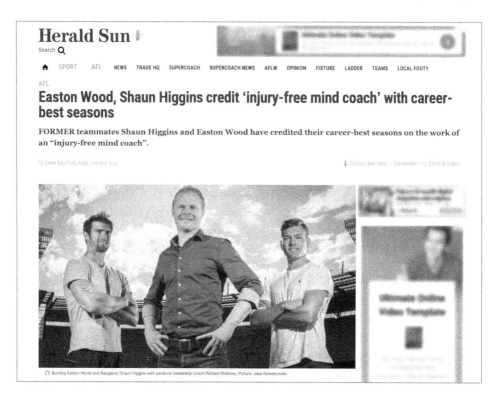

realised I needed to coach more people remotely in real time, and this is when the QM program really began to evolve, via the introduction of the mobile phone app.

In the last three years, I've finally refined the Quality Mind program and app to exactly where they need to be, and I'm thrilled to say that this business is now my full time passion and my full time career. I have been amazed by the extraordinary results and the growth that we are achieving, and I can now say with surety that I am living my true purpose. This book will take you on quite the journey, but I implore you to stick with it, and I promise you that if you do, your life will change for the better!

Enjoy the ride!

The Quality Mind Model

Quality Mind's core model is based on modern day science and is a blend of

- Practices of Neuroscience
- Practices of Positive Psychology
- Practices of Neuro Linguistic Programming (NLP)
- Knowledge of HeartMath Institute
- Practices of Ancient Philosophies

Neuroscience (or neurobiology) is the scientific study of the nervous system. It is the branch of biology that investigates the molecular, cellular, developmental, functional, evolutionary, computational, psychosocial and medical aspects of the brain. It's very scientific, but we break it down for you throughout the book, in layman's terms!

Positive Psychology is the scientific study of the strengths that enable individuals and communities to thrive. The field is founded on the belief that people want to lead meaningful and fulfilling lives, to cultivate what is best within themselves, and to enhance their experiences of love, work, and play.

Neuro-Linguistic Programming (NLP) is a way of communicating, created in the 1970s. It is often shortened to NLP. NLP is all about bringing about changes in perception, responsible communication and developing choices of responses or communication in a given situation. NLP works on the principle that everyone has all the resources they need to make positive changes in their own life. I am a trained Master NLP Practitioner.

HeartMath technology is the most influential part of our program, and it is an innovative approach to improving emotional wellbeing. It teaches you to change your heart rhythm pattern to create physiological coherence, a scientifically measurable state characterized by increased order and harmony in our mind, emotions and body. I am a certified HeartMath trainer.

Ancient Philosophies: the ability to think and act using knowledge, experience, understanding, common sense and insight. Wisdom is associated with attributes such as unbiased judgment, compassion, experiential self-knowledge, self-transcendence and non-attachment, and virtues such as ethics and benevolence.

The QM multi-level system eliminates life's challenges by using smart phone technology and trained Mind Mentors™ to reduce the likelihood and severity of injuries, illness and burnout.

We are balancing and connecting people to their intuition and pointing them in the right direction. When you are fully plugged into the NOW and racing toward your highest excitement, anything is possible. This book will push all levels of understanding, education, and mainstream psychology as we dive into an understanding of reality and our relationship to life that is radically beyond today's widely expected and accepted life experience. We'll do all of this with practical mental training that will help you to elevate yourself to your next level or bring you back in line with the athlete you've always been, no matter the sport you play.

As you read through this book, AND TAKE MASSIVE ACTION, it will recode you to a higher understanding, get rid of the default programs clogging up your mind, and wake you up to the true (and better) version of yourself. The one who moves through life and sport the way you were always meant to — effortlessly, consistent in performance and free of injury.

Now Download the Quality Mind App

Before reading any further, it's time for you to pick up your mobile phone and download the Quality Mind app to your iOS or Android device. Simply head into the App Store or Google Play, search for "Quality Mind Global," and you'll be on your way. It's free, or you can upgrade to the Premium level.

The Quality Mind program is highly interactive and you'll find that the app is the best friend you could have in your pocket along this journey. This book was written to be used alongside and in unison with the phone / iPad app. The book will put you on the right path, while the app will keep you accountable to the learning as well as grounded and connected to the community along the way.

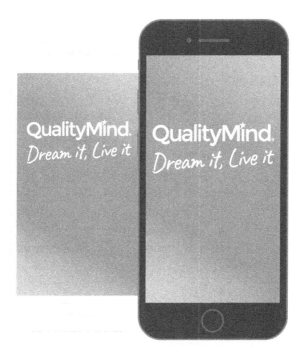

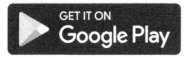 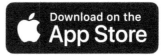

Key Areas

Each of these terms will be explored in more depth later in the book; however, since you'll see them right away in the app, we'll go ahead and give you a cheat sheet.

Thought Shopping: This is the most frequently used tool in the app and it will keep you aware of where your mind and feelings are throughout the day. When you notice you're in a negative space, use personalised triggers to disrupt your thinking and feeling, and to elevate your energy.

Bubble Popping: Limiting beliefs and life's everyday obstacles are a fact of life, but they don't have to be. Bubble Popping is a self-coaching tool that allows you to remove harmful 'deeper' challenges that are holding you back, and then supports you as you process and dissolve them. Remember the thought bubbles above the heads of our most loved comic book characters growing up? Well, your thought goes in a bubble much like that — you work through the questions, and then you pop it to eliminate the issue. It's very satisfying!

Meditation & Relaxation: Meditation is a form of deep relaxation that enables you to stay in the moment and connect to your innate awareness. The cool thing about the Quality Mind app is that it comes loaded with hundreds of guided, non-guided and walking meditations of various lengths, with different areas of focus, from beginners through advanced — from those that promote deep sleep and pain relief, to a post-performance routine, to unleashing your creativity. It also offers ambient lounge music and science-based music with binaural beats (also known as sound wave therapy) offering multiple frequency levels to cater for every situation and mood. We're adding more all the time from experts around the world.

My Journal: A journey is often most appreciated and most productive when we utilise a dedicated space to share our thoughts and reflections. This introspective space in the app encourages you to tell your story and share your discoveries with yourself. All clients who opt to access personal mentoring will also be able to chat to their Mind Mentor in real time via the Journal in the app.

Body Balance: Sports medicine is an elite science, and every pro athlete is in capable hands managing their physical form. It helps with motivation and accountability when one has a dedicated place to record daily physical activity — from high intensity interval training to yoga to elite training. It's also a place where you can keep a food journal.

Reminders & Notifications: If you want to change your life, all you need to do, quite simply, is change your behaviors. In this section, you'll be able to program your daily reminders, alerting you that it's time to activate your Quality Mind. Initially, we recommend hourly reminders for optimal change, and this is always our default setting. You do have the ability to adjust this, however, to the intervals that best suit you.

Now that you've downloaded the app, registered your account, and acquainted yourself with its key areas, you're ready to proceed!

Introduction

Are you an athlete playing at any level of sport, striving for the best game, the best form, and the best career possible? If so, this book is for you. Whether you're playing in the AFL, the NFL, the NBA, UFC, or FIFA, not to mention all the other renowned sports organizations around the world, *Injury-Free* can help you become a better athlete, manager and coach.

The Quality Mind program is for athletes training for the Olympics, for professional players (both retired or current), or even for someone just trying to improve their golf game. It's designed to provide maximum benefits for anyone wanting to improve their life. If you sense this invisible but very real gap between how you're playing and how you want to play, either in sport or in life, this book will help you — providing you follow my step-by-step system. And it's not just for the individual — entire organizations can team up and go on the Quality Mind journey together.

Now that you've got this self-directed Personal Activation System in your hands and the app on your smartphone, you're ready to get started!

The first step toward a Quality Mind is becoming aware of the control you have over your own mind. The truth is that in many ways our minds are like puppies! Everyone loves a puppy; they're adorable and we watch entirely too many videos of them on YouTube. When you first bring a puppy home, you welcome it into the house and let it run wild. It's fine at first. So cute! No problem. Within a day or two, however, the house stinks and the furniture's been ripped apart because the new dog doesn't know how to act or where to do its business. This is basically what happens with our minds! Without adequate training, the mind just races around in so many unproductive directions, making a mess and never getting anything done. When each day's thoughts are 90% repetitive of the thoughts we had in the days before, it's no surprise that we lose critical energy and focus from circular, self-defeating thought patterns.

So, how do we change that? The same way we get the puppy to change: through training. When the dog's running amok and making a mess, you leash the dog, put it in its own space, and clean your house up. Then you bring the dog back inside to play when it's appropriate. The puppy grows into an obedient dog who adds value to the household. By the same token, your undisciplined mind grows into a purposeful mind, and that mind is in full control of itself. You step into the coaches box, and you actually become the coach of your own life. The best coaches are watching the game from the outside in, and you will become that coach. You'll be a spectator of your own mind, allowing you to see things with clarity and from a more controlled and analytical perspective.

Unfortunately, as many athletes are now understanding and appreciating, when the mind is not firing well or with clarity, the synchronised body will reflect this more often than not. This heavily impacts sports performance and team success, so let's now look at the latest data and the cost to teams when the body breaks down.

What is the Real Cost of Injuries in Professional Sport?

We all know that injuries are a huge and costly problem in sport today, and we also know that they are on the rise. Nobody likes to see athletes injured, and we understand that teams are negatively affected when they are without their best talent, but do we really understand how much injuries truly affect teams?

When we think about the salaries paid to elite athletes today, it's pretty easy to grasp that it's a huge financial drain on an organisation when an athlete is injured and teams have millions of dollars sitting on the bench. According to Kitmanlabs[2], over $700,000,000 was spent on salaries for injured athletes in Major League Baseball (MLB) in 2015, over $450,000,000 in the National Football League (NFL), $350,000,000 in the National Basketball Association (NBA) and $300,000,000 in the English Premier League.

However, we also know the effect of injuries extends far beyond the monetary impact on a team. When thinking about sports at its purest level, only one thing really matters..... WINNING. And sadly, this is often the REAL COST of injury. It's the difference between winning and losing.

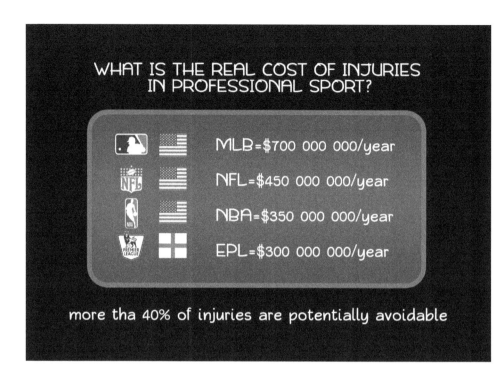

Given that we know injuries are preventable and that there are numerous modifiable risk factors, this gives rise to the importance of appropriate management and the use of analytics — not just to showcase the problem, but to solve it. Kitmanlabs[2] also reported that over 40% of injuries in the NFL are potentially avoidable. That's not just a marginal gain, that's a game changer. And the missing link and the critical growth area is the UNTAPPED MIND.

In Australia, sport injury (both semiprofessional and professional), costs the economy around $2 billion a year, which is on par with obesity, widely regarded as one of the nation's biggest public health challenges. Rather significant, wouldn't you say?!

2. https://www.kitmanlabs.com/what-is-the-real-cost-of-injuries-in-professional-sport/

The 5 Key Areas Where Athletes Break Down

The key to being *Injury-Free* is continuously becoming self-aware by connecting to your **heart space** and getting in touch moment by moment with your innate **intuition**, and then letting life flow to you. If you're not feeling love, compassion, happiness, and appreciation, then you're in your Child's mind (I will explain). That's not the place you want to be — you create your own reality, so existing in worry and fear will simply create more fear and worry. Sound simple? Yes it is, with practice!

As an elite athlete, your highest excitement is often performing on the big stage, entertaining the crowds, and dominating the play. When you become worried or fearful of what other people think, or whether something's going to happen, you get out of alignment with your true potential. And when you get lost in fear, you lose touch with your true self. This is where you will run in to trouble and possibly manifest a breakdown.

"The body is led by the mind"

#1. Not unconditionally excited

If you are not fully excited and whole-heartedly invested in the opportunity that has been offered to you, or if you are only seeing the benefits and the personal gains that come with the job, then you are putting yourself in jeopardy. This is when breakdowns can, and most likely will occur. The opposite of excitement is carrying elements of fear (as mentioned above), and in order to follow your highest excitement, you must first identify and understand your PURPOSE, or your WHY in life. If you live by your purpose (e.g. to inspire youth, to demonstrate your skills on the big stage as an influencer of the community, or simply to help or make other people happy), then the stars will align and you will achieve success.

As soon as you lose the love for the game, the game will lose its love for you. If you're not feeling the love, then read on, and this book will show you how to turn that around.

#2. Not 100% Focussed

When an athlete is not 110% focused on their direction of success, that lack of focus can cause a breakdown and will cause inconsistencies in performance. "Where your focus goes, your energy flows."

There are a million things you could be distracted by — perhaps you've got a new partner, or retirement is fast approaching. Maybe you've just had a baby, or there's a business opportunity you're thinking about, or media commitments are consuming your focus? Or maybe you're always blaming others for your not being selected in the team? Whatever the distraction, if you're not 110% focused on maximising your talent, you could find yourself being injured or omitted from the team due to poor performance. That's not something you can blame on the coach or the organization.

Another common challenge for athletes is managing the 'second year blues'. A lot of athletes will have a standout season when they first join the team, but then find their second year performance is well below their standard. Think about what's changed here. It's the athletes mindset, excitement levels and focus. It's all you, and you need to own that in order to address it and resolve it.

Finally, when your focus is not where it should be, your Child's mind can ambush and make stupid and/or childish decisions. For example: emotional or aggressive outbursts, blowing off steam with substance abuse and rash decisions that are not well thought out and can lead to a tarnished reputation or injury.

#3. Lacking Self-Worth (which is a fear)

If you have low feelings of self-worth and regularly beat yourself up, you are heading for a breakdown. Constantly judging yourself and putting yourself down undermines your entire self. How can you reach your dreams and achieve your goals when you fundamentally believe that you don't deserve them? This sort of thinking will take you on a downward spiral. And as your inner feelings of worthlessness affect your performance on the field, the path of injury will become inevitable and unavoidable.

If you lack self-worth and you don't believe in yourself, you won't be able to reach peak performance and fire consistently at the top level. My process gives you the tools and awareness to define and illuminate these areas in your life so that you can consistently play to the absolute best of your ability.

When kids get to the elite sport level, a large percentage of them don't have the mental capacity to consistently compete at those levels. Their body may be strong and professionally managed, but their minds are not. They need a reliable process to recognize how to clean out their mental filters of everyday junk, get in flow with life, and become receptive to life's bounty — which includes reaching and realizing their dreams and creating their own reality.

#4. Harboring Repeating Fears

If you have any element of man-made fear repeating inside you, that fear is going to manifest in your reality and you're a big chance to get injured. This includes fear of the future — are you going to perform in your next game? Or fear of the past — are you going to make the same mistakes again? It could be fear of success, and all of the expectations that come with it, or fear of not being successful and never embodying your potential, or fear of being found out. These are just a few examples, and fear tends to spiral and gain momentum. The more you fear, the more you fear.

Just know this — whatever fear you are feeling, is UNNECESSARY! Your **heart-mind** (more on this ahead) already knows how to take you where you want to go. Allow life to flow to you with an open heart, and please don't get in your own way!

#5. Not Listening To Your Body — Fatigue

Most elite sports scientists today are on the cutting edge and they are collecting comprehensive extensive data to monitor workload stress levels (both on and off the field) to the point where every minute is analyzed and the statistical probability of injury is consistently measured to determine when an athlete should be rested. This is progressive and effective at times; however, nothing beats the intuition we experience when we are in complete balance and alignment with who we are. When our minds are in perfect coherence, we easily recognise and acknowledge the inner alarm bells in the body, and we understand when to take note, and when to push through. This innate intuition needs to be tapped in to though, and there is an art to understanding how to access it. You will always be the ultimate judge of your capabilities, but if you're not appropriately connected or balanced, then your intuition will be off and your ego will most likely overshadow this inner GPS signal.

The Quality Mind process offers a solution to these 5 key concerns, and I'm ready to spill our secrets. Now are you ready to get everything you've ever wanted?

Athlete Timeline Example — Your Time is Short

If you look at the history of many elite athletes, you'll discover that nine times out of ten they are injury free up until a certain point, or most of them are playing consistent sport until a certain point — and that point is usually when pressure has been applied and a mental shift occurs. Then they move from playing for excitement to playing in fear or playing it safe. This is key.

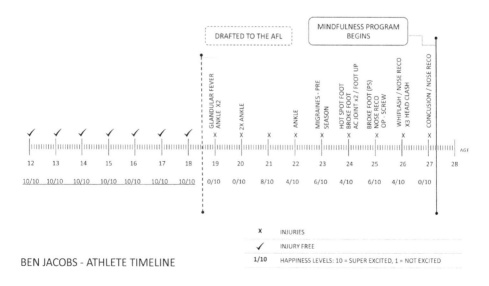

BEN JACOBS - ATHLETE TIMELINE

Ben Jacobs Self Assessed Life & Sports Timeline

Once athletes begin to recognize their recurring patterns of thought and access a logical understanding of how they feel, it can shed some light on what is going on in their lives, such as why and when they've suffered certain types of injuries and performance issues. We can map these out for our athletes with a timeline diagram. For our AFL players for example, we often track their career from age 12, or whenever they started playing football before they went pro.

Let's take a look at the athlete timeline for Ben Jacobs, a 27-year-old AFL player with North Melbourne Football Club (page 27).

I start with following the athlete's age on the horizontal axis. With Ben, we began tracking his overall excitement for playing the game from 12 years old. Throughout his junior years, his excitement was maxed out, 10/10, and he played without injury. No pressure.

Throughout the junior years of most AFL athletes, between 12 to 15 years of age, they may have a couple of minor injuries — but more often than not, they don't. If they do have injuries that are consistent, that usually means their self-worth has been compromised during that time and they have some limiting beliefs that they're already carrying around with them.

For determined athletes with elite potential, they'll usually go through that period injury-free. They often won't start to feel the pressure until they're being watched by recruiters, which happens between the ages of 16 and 20.

What you see on Ben's timeline is that the injuries occur when the pressure comes on. Something has happened in the external world that causes the internal world to crack. For Ben, it was his recruitment to the AFL. His excitement playing the game plummeted, both caused by and causing various injuries. He's injured his ankles multiple times, faced nose reconstruction twice, and is currently dealing with the aftermath of concussion. Because Ben didn't have the Quality Mind toolkit, external pressures intensified his inner turmoil, until injury resulted and the cycle began again, compounded by what came before.

Ben Jacobs Case Study

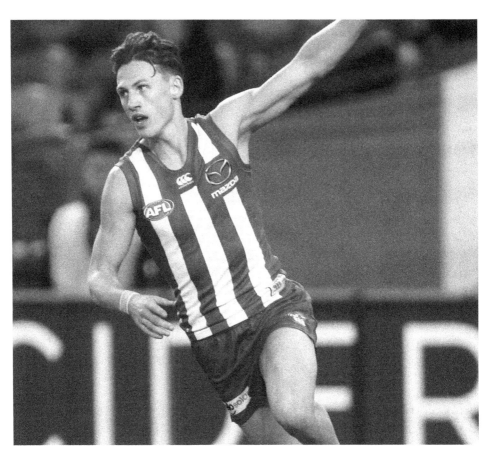

Ben Jacobs, North Melbourne FC Player (AFL) — Courtesy AFL Photos

Ben Jacobs grew up in the bayside suburb of Beaumaris, Victoria, Australia. He developed a passion for Australian Rules Football from a very young age, and at that time he also developed a very clear and unwavering goal to get drafted to the AFL. He had no doubt this would happen, so no- one was surprised when he was Port Adelaide FC's first selection and the 16th overall selection in the 2010 Australian Football League National Draft. He is known for his excellent marking and ball winning ability, with great core strength and the ability to run all day.

Unfortunately, Ben was sidelined due to concussion in round 16 last season (2018) and he has yet to fully recover, dealing with serious and ongoing concussion related trauma. Whilst he is still on the sideline, he is doing everything possible to get himself back on the ground for the 2020 AFL season. Ben's story offers an honest and eye-opening message about balancing the mind/body connection and the importance of understanding how stress impacts both on and off the field, if not managed well.

We asked Ben, "What would your advice be for young up and coming athletes, and for your younger self"?

"My advice would definitely be to go back to the pure enjoyment of the game. I don't look back and go geez, I wish I had worked harder, because I was already working hard and still continue to do so. I just wish I had enjoyed my time more coming through as a new recruit, because you don't know when it's going to end, and you take it all for granted. I wish I had enjoyed every little moment more, even the challenge of a setback, instead of beating myself up. So, this is what I work on doing now!"

"A lot of the time in speeches of past elite athletes and current team leaders I hear them saying, you're only going to be playing for a short amount of time so make the most of it, like, just work extra hard. But I don't look at it like that anymore. My advice would be completely different. My advice would be — you're only in it a short time, so make sure you enjoy it. And I think if you're enjoying something, you're going to do your best in it naturally anyway. For me, looking back there was definitely a pattern, which I have now fixed. When I enjoyed it, that's when I just played the best footy, you know? And just let go of all the other rubbish."

We asked Ben, "What have you learned about yourself since you've been involved with Quality Mind"?

"Thankfully with Quality Mind I've had a total perspective change on everything in life. I'm just really enjoying and loving the transition in my awareness, and getting that balance between knowing you've got goals, but also just living in the now and trusting yourself and the process. I've learned patience, and that's probably one of the main things. Sure, I've got goals, but you can actually get in the way of your goals if you're constantly worrying, stressing and beating yourself up over it. It's a totally new and invigorating mindset, and just a game changer for me."

So Ben, would you recommend Quality Mind?

"Yes. 100%! I think it's a must for any aspiring athlete, and just anyone in general. I'm a total advocate, and I'm always talking to people around me about it and they're now trying to implement the QM techniques as well. Luckily, I'm only 27 and I've still got years ahead of me. And what I now love to do is pass this amazing knowledge along because I think it's a must, especially for the young ones that can just completely avoid all that worry and pain and injury."

For a more intimate look into what this cycle looks like, let's take a deeper look into my own past. When I was a young football player, I was regularly featured in the best players list in my competition, and I was always that kid that was possibly going to be drafted by an elite team. Even at the age of 12, the local newspaper wrote me up as 'one to watch'.

But then when I finally got there, I didn't have the adequate mental foundation needed to consistently succeed. I'd simply always been the one of the best, and I didn't have a great attitude or work ethic because I had always achieved what I needed to without discipline. Plus, I wasn't 100% committed to my future, and my mind was like an untrained puppy!

Throughout my adolescent years, I dealt with bouts of anxiety and difficult life situations, mainly through my decision making. At the age of 18, my parents separated, as I said, which added additional pressure to my life. I broke my thumb and had ongoing back issues that fed into hamstring injuries and related pain. I also used to break my ribs a lot. It was a really difficult time!

For many athletes, the pressure goes on, then the mind starts to crack, then the body follows suit. It's usually a predictable and cyclical process, and it's difficult to halt. If you're feeling a lack of self-worth, low confidence, or are afraid of making mistakes, then the body will hear the constant negativity that's flowing through your mind and shut down to pull you out of that extreme situation. Remember, the mind's role is to keep you safe (more on this soon).

Many athletes become trapped in their own minds and they can feel their excitement levels decreasing, which means they're not playing on

SPORT
OCTOBER 7, 1987

On track for the Saints!

THE football season has ended, but there is just one thing on the mind of 12-year-old Richard Maloney, St Francis Junior Football Club's star player.

Richard, who lives at Beaumaris, wants to play VFL football with St Kilda, and there are no prizes for guessing that Tony Lockett is his favorite player.

The little dynamo's success on the field this year has been remarkable.

31 votes

Playing in the Under-12 Chelsea Districts junior football competition, Richard was selected as the best player in the grand final, won the league best and fairest with an incredible 31 votes, represented VFA club Sandringham in a match against Ballarat, represented St Francis in a Chelsea Districts combined side, and won the club best and fairest.

Not even Tony Lockett could match that!

Richard's father, Peter Maloney, said his son had been winning a similar number of awards each season for the past three years.

"He has a natural talent for the game, but he eats and sleeps football anyway," he said.

Last year Richard won the best and fairest award for the St Kilda Little League side and has won, or was runner-up in, best and fairest awards in the Chelsea Districts competition since his games in the Under-10s.

More recently he was runner-up in the best and fairest in his Under-13 school football team at Mentone Grammar School.

"Richard plays in the centre and as a ruck rover, but I think he will turn out a Brad Hardy type of player," said his father, who is also team manager of the St Francis Under-12s.

— LES HAMS.

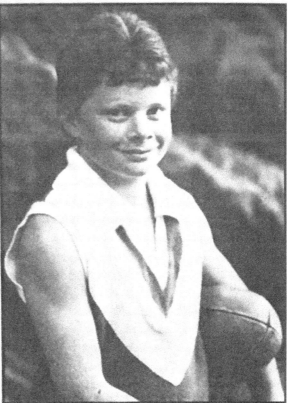

CHAMPION junior footballer Richard Maloney ... hopes to play for St Kilda.

Richard Maloney featuring in the local newspaper, October 7, 1987 natural flow energy anymore. They are now playing from a place of fear, which drains their energy and gets them worried about the future or past. This eliminates an athlete's *now* factor, and they're suddenly playing their sport whilst constantly thinking. They are not in the moment, and therefore they are out of flow.

The elite sports system today struggles to manage the mental health of their players. Many top draft picks regularly break down, either mentally or physically, because of the level of pressure from the media, the club's marketing strategies, the general public, and everyone's expectations. Young athletes can't handle it all because their minds haven't been built with a strong foundation, which needs to flow back to our educational system and our guidance. We're just not adequately educated or equipped these days, both here in Australia and globally. This issue is by no means confined to sport either — we are facing a global crisis when it comes to mental health.

When we see that a player's performance is inconsistent and is continuously going up and down, up and down, it's generally because there is no continuity of the mind. The excitement is wavering, the pressure is on and fears are cementing. And when you get to the elite level, there are multiple experts pressuring you to get your diet in check, behave appropriately, make sure you know the playbook, attend media functions, sign merchandise, and so on and so on. These kids do their best, but they're usually no longer sleeping well. Their thoughts become repetitive, and those thoughts then solidify into limiting beliefs. Next thing they're heading down a troubling track of inconsistent play, which only exacerbates their inner turmoil. Their minds become clogged with unproductive and stressful thoughts and feelings, like mind sludge that weighs them down further and further.

In today's professional sporting world, an athlete should be treated like a Ferrari engine being tended to by a Formula One racing team. When the Ferrari's initial warning lights flash on the dashboard, the driver or engineer immediately pulls the Ferrari off the track to give it a closer look, and the first place they look is under the hood.

Unfortunately, though, the majority of our sports coaches, scientists, and even our psychologists, are not adequately equipped to recognize when this elusive warning light is flashing on the dashboard of an elite athlete. And they're not getting close enough to see what's really happening under the hood. When they do finally notice, it's often too late because the athlete has already crashed.

In the world of elite sports, the coaches, sports scientists, psychologists etc. are all first-rate; however, many times, they have no idea why athletes are breaking down. The reality is that these young athletes are being led by their mind, which hasn't been armed with the strong foundation necessary for peak play. Catching the thought patterns that contribute to this decline in health and form is crucial, but it is not something sports experts are currently able to recognize. This is where the Quality Mind app comes in. It allows sports scientists, psychologists, coaches, managers and the rest of us to identify when the "needs service" light goes on in an athlete's mind. It helps the athlete recognize and address it too, providing they use the app multiple times a day with complete honesty. Otherwise, neither they nor we have the data required to help them. We will show you more of these timelines as we journey forward together.

Intelligent Energy Management

One of the most important steps in being able to prevent energy drains and increase resilience is to expand our awareness and identify unnecessary energy expenditures.

Resilience, optimal performance, fulfillment and health are grounded in our intelligent management of energy expenditures and our ability to renew energy.

Depleting Your Energy

Emotions such as fear, frustration, impatience and anger evoke a toxic feeling and cause the release of stress hormones.

This often results in:

- Reduced muscle mass
- Brain-cell death
- Impaired memory
- Accelerated aging
- Impaired mental function
- Diminished performance

Renewing Your Energy

Emotions and attitudes such as care, courage, tolerance and appreciation create neurochemicals that regenerate your system and offset energy drain, resulting in:

- Increased longevity
- Increased resilience to adversity

- Improved memory
- Improved problem-solving
- Increased intuition and creativity
- Improved job performance and achievement

Reaching the next level of athletic performance depends upon your ability to regulate emotions and manage stress. Athletes who combine mental and emotional training with their physical training have a competitive advantage and are better equipped to enter into the peak performance zone more consistently.

Thoughts and emotions have a profound effect on the heart's rhythm, and this rhythm impacts performance. Under pressure, stressful thoughts and emotions cause the heart's rhythm to become irregular and jagged. This incoherent pattern inhibits brain function, diminishes the visual field, reduces reaction speed and impairs decision making.

Conversely, a positive mental and emotional state, not unlike being 'in the zone,' creates a smooth, wave-like, coherent pattern that facilitates brain function and improves mental focus and physical coordination.

Let's take a deeper look into this via modern-day science.

Home Is Where The Heart Is

New scientific research shows the human heart is much more than an efficient pump that sustains life. Research suggests the heart is also an access point to a source of wisdom and intelligence that we can call upon to live our lives with more balance, greater creativity, and enhanced intuitive capacities. All of these are important for increasing personal effectiveness, improving health and relationships and achieving greater fulfillment.

The Intelligent Heart

The following few pages provide a deep dive into modern day science. This information provides further proof and academic validation that what we are offering in this book is more than just a hunch or an opinion. It's fact. It's modern science, and it's necessary for us to share. In saying that, it is science none the less, so if it's too much for your brain to decipher, feel free to skip through to page 42!

Many of the changes in bodily functions that occur during the coherent state revolve around changes in the heart's pattern of activity. While the heart is certainly a remarkable pump, interestingly, it is only relatively recently in the course of human history — in the past three centuries or so — that the heart's function has been defined (by Western scientific thought) as only that of pumping blood. Historically, in almost every culture around the world, the heart was ascribed a far more multifaceted role in the human system, regarded as a source of wisdom, spiritual insight, thought and emotion. Intriguingly, scientific research over the past several decades has begun to provide evidence that many of these long-surviving associations may well be more than simply metaphorical. These developments have led science to once again revise and expand its understanding of the heart and the role of this amazing organ.

In the new field of neurocardiology, for example, scientists have discovered that the heart possesses its own intrinsic nervous system—a network of nerves so functionally sophisticated as to earn the description of a "heart brain." Containing over 40,000 neurons, this "little brain" gives the heart the ability to independently sense, process information, make decisions, and even to demonstrate a type of learning and memory. In essence, it appears that the heart is truly an intelligent system. Research has also revealed that the heart is a hormonal gland, manufacturing and secreting numerous hormones and neurotransmitters that profoundly affect brain and body function. Among the hormones the heart produces is oxytocin — well known as the "love" or "bonding hormone." Science has only begun to understand the effects of the electromagnetic fields produced by the heart, but there is evidence that the information contained in the heart's powerful field may play a vital synchronizing role in the human body — and that it may affect others around us as well.

Research has also shown that the heart is a key component of the emotional system. Scientists now understand that the heart not only responds to emotion, but that the signals generated by its rhythmic activity actually play a major part in determining the quality of our emotional experience from moment to moment. As described next, these heart signals also profoundly impact perception and cognitive function by virtue of the heart's extensive communication network with the brain. Finally, rigorous electrophysiological studies conducted at the HeartMath Institute have even indicated that the heart appears to play a key role in intuition. Although there is much yet to be understood, it appears that the age-old associations of the heart with thought, feeling and insight may indeed have a basis in science.

The heart has been considered the source of emotion, courage and wisdom for centuries. For more than 25 years, the HeartMath Institute Research Center has explored the physiological mechanisms by which the heart and brain communicate and how the activity of the heart influences our perceptions, emotions, intuition and health. Early on in their research they asked, among other questions, why people experience the feeling or sensation of love and other regenerative emotions as well as heartache in the physical area of the heart.

In the early 1990s, they were among the first to conduct research that not only looked at how stressful emotions affect activity in the autonomic nervous system (ANS) and the hormonal and immune systems, but also at the effects of emotions such as appreciation, compassion and care.

It became clear that stressful or depleting emotions such as frustration and overwhelming emotions lead to increased disorder in the higher-level brain centers and autonomic nervous system. These are reflected in the heart rhythms and adversely affect the functioning of virtually all bodily systems. This eventually led to a much deeper understanding of the neural and other communication pathways between the heart and brain. They also observed that the *heart acted as though it had a mind of its own* and could significantly influence the way we perceive and respond in our daily interactions. In essence, it appeared that the heart could affect our awareness, perceptions and intelligence. Numerous studies have since shown that heart coherence is an optimal physiological state associated with increased cognitive function, self-regulatory capacity, emotional stability, and resilience.

The Heart-Brain Connection

Most of us have been taught in school that the heart is constantly responding to "orders" sent by the brain in the form of neural signals. However, it is not as commonly known that:

- In fetal development, the heart forms and begins beating before the brain begins to develop.

- The heart can continue to function without any connection to a functioning brain.
- The heart actually sends more communication to the brain than the brain sends to the heart!

Moreover, these heart signals have a significant effect on brain function — influencing emotional processing as well as higher cognitive faculties such as attention, perception, memory, and problem-solving. In other words, not only does the heart respond to the brain, but the brain continuously responds to the heart.

The effect of heart activity on brain function has been researched extensively over the past 40 years. Earlier research mainly examined the effects of heart activity occurring on a very short time scale — over several consecutive heartbeats at maximum. Scientists have extended this body of scientific research by looking at how larger-scale patterns of heart activity affect the brain's functioning.

Their research has demonstrated that different patterns of heart activity (which accompany different emotional states) have distinct effects on cognitive and emotional function. During stress and negative emotions, when the heart rhythm pattern is erratic and disordered, the corresponding pattern of neural signals traveling from the heart to the brain inhibits higher cognitive functions.

This limits our ability to think clearly, remember, learn, reason, and make effective decisions. (This helps explain why we may often act impulsively and unwisely when we're under stress.) The heart's input to the brain during stressful or negative emotions also has a profound effect on the brain's emotional processes — actually serving to reinforce the emotional experience of stress.

In contrast, the more ordered and stable pattern of the heart's input to the brain during positive emotional states has the opposite effect — it facilitates cognitive function and reinforces positive feelings and emotional stability. This means that learning to generate increased heart rhythm coherence, by sustaining positive emotions, not only benefits the entire body but also profoundly affects how we perceive, think, feel, and perform as an athlete.

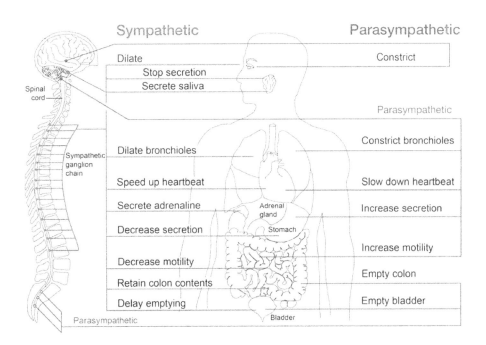

Image courtesy of the HeartMath® Institute — www.heartmath.org

The Autonomic Nervous System (ANS) regulates 90% of the body's internal processes, including breathing, heart rate, digestion, immune system, important aspects of the hormonal system, alertness and sleep.

The ANS has two branches which both connect to the heart: the sympathetic and parasympathetic. When these are out of sync with each other, it can be likened to driving a car with one foot on the gas pedal (the sympathetic nervous system) and the other on the brake (the parasympathetic nervous system) at the same time — this creates a jerky ride, burns more gas, and isn't great for your car, either! Likewise, the incoherent patterns of physiological activity associated with stressful emotions can cause our body to operate inefficiently, deplete our energy, and produce extra wear and tear on our whole system. This is especially true if stress and negative emotions are prolonged or experienced often.

In contrast, positive, renewing emotions send a very different signal throughout our body. When we experience uplifting feelings such as appreciation, joy, care and love, our heart rhythm pattern becomes highly ordered, looking like a smooth, harmonious wave (an example is shown in the figure below). This is called a coherent heart rhythm pattern. When we are generating a coherent heart rhythm, the activity in the two branches of the ANS is synchronized and the body's systems operate with increased efficiency and harmony. It's no wonder that positive emotions feel so good — they actually help our body's systems synchronize and work better.

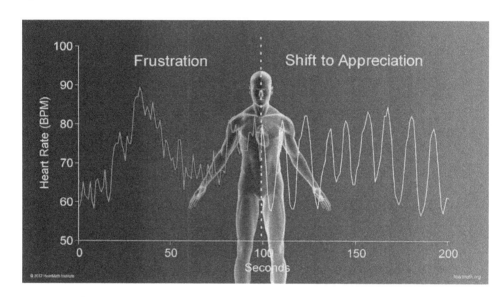

Image courtesy of the HeartMath® Institute — www.heartmath.org

Coherence: A State of Peak Performance

Research has shown that generating sustained positive emotions facilitates a body-wide shift to a specific, scientifically measurable state. This state is termed psychophysiological coherence because it is characterized by increased order and harmony in both our psychological (mental and emotional) and physiological (bodily) processes. Psychophysiological coherence is a state of optimal function. Research shows that when we activate this state, our physiological systems function more efficiently, we experience greater emotional stability, and we also have increased mental clarity and improved cognitive function. Simply stated, our body and brain work better, we feel better, and we perform better.

And for athletes, these are a few of the benefits of being heart focussed.

- Maximum concentration, focus and mental clarity — even under pressure
- Improved motor coordination and reaction time speeds; reduced muscle tremors (yips)
- Perceptual clarity for better decision making on and off the field/course
- Team coherence — increased intuitive synchronization with other team members
- Self-regulation of fear, performance anxiety, worry and frustration

In summary, the one with the most energy wins the race, and we've discovered that we all have the ability to tap into new reservoirs of energy from within, — via the heart. We actually have superpowers (in the form of energy) that lie dormant within the human structure. We've all seen examples of this — such as when someone is trapped in or under a car after an accident and their rescuer somehow manages to lift an entire car, with no understanding of how on earth they were able to do it. This super energy cannot just be called upon, it's pure heart at work and it will only emerge when you are pure heart, and when you are 100% in the moment. More on this ahead!

Information Courtesy of the HeartMath Institute, where Richard Maloney is a Certified HeartMath Trainer — www.heartmath.org

The Five Steps To Creating a Quality Mind

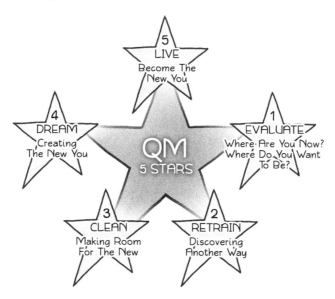

The Steps to create a 5 Star 'Quality' Life

We live in the age of information, and most of us now have access to the world and all its knowledge, thanks to technology, which has closed the proverbial gap. In the past, the lion's share of knowledge was in the hands of those in authoritarian roles or those with money and power, and there was a separation between those people and the masses. Today, however, even the teachings from ancient philosophers are now widely available and accepted, and with the answers to just about everything at our fingertips, people are becoming more knowledgeable and more informed.

With this new access to information and knowledge, we are experiencing an increase in awareness — and awareness is consciousness. So we are now seeing a strong, fundamental change in the way people are interacting in their environment, and in the world. Quite simply, people are waking up!

What was considered cutting edge just a few years ago may now be considered obsolete, or will already have been superseded. We see examples of this every day. For instance, just look at your parents' mobile phones. They're just so 2015! The world today is moving far more rapidly than ever before because of technology, and, in turn, everybody's gaining information at speeds we've never seen before.

Consequently, we are now seeing the economy, politics, religious models, medical models, the environment and education all showing consistent cracks because the old models can't sustain themselves in these rapidly changing and evolving times. People are beginning to realize that it's not enough to just know, and that this is the time in history to know 'how'.

If I look back to ten years ago when I was selling and teaching meditation to government departments and corporate business, I was seen as somewhat of a 'tree hugger'. It was such a tough sell back then, and even once we were in, it was almost impossible to get the majority of our clients to immerse themselves in our program. They simply didn't understand or accept the concept of meditation and its benefits, and it was considered too left field for most people to embrace it. Thankfully today, things are very different. Meditation went from hippy to hobby, and today it's now recognised as a 'critical' factor in many organisations globally.

There is still a general resistance to people really working deeply on themselves, however, this is definitely changing as technology evolves and open discussions about mental health become more commonplace. In fact, in my opinion, it will soon become recognised as both cool and critical to shed your mental garbage, and this will start with our leaders and filter down. Leaders today require more than just knowledge and experience. They must gain higher levels of self-awareness and demonstrate authentic levels of inner intelligence. When our leaders show how connected they are to their true selves, we will then see a paradigm shift in consciousness, and this really excites me!

What I am seeing today is more and more people with the desire to invest in learning how to apply their growth areas, advance their behaviors and self-awareness, and do something differently. There is a deep inner yearning emerging for many, and this yearning creates the need for new experiences. One of the wonderful things about new experiences is that they enrich the circuitry in the brain, and as a side effect of this change in circuitry, we begin to experience happiness and light.

If you provide people with new opportunities to connect with and advance themselves, and you apply the science in a way that is easy to understand and repeat on a regular basis, then you're really getting somewhere. In the case of Quality Mind, we help people to recondition their minds and bodies via the repetitive use of our very simple and effective mobile phone app. Over time, you will neuro-chemically recondition your mind, body and soul to work as one, and once you reach that point, it starts to become a state of being.

People then go from defaulting to their over thinking 'Child' mind to utilising their 'Master' mind, which is life changing! I watch people go from knowledge, to experience, to the incredible 2.0 version of themselves when this takes place. From mind to body to soul. From thinking to doing to being. From acting to becoming. From applying with practice, to then knowing by heart. Then, the personal advances and changes take full effect.

Once you begin to think differently, you feel differently, and then you do differently, and that can quite literally alter what's happening in your nervous system, in your circulatory system and in your body. I've personally witnessed clients heal themselves of cancer, and we've seen clients throw away their anxiety medications in just a few weeks. The information alone, however, is not enough. You have to close the gap between knowledge and experience and take meaningful, authentic, accountable daily action. This is why I have designed the Quality Mind process around elements of neuroscience, positive psychology, heartmath technology, NLP and ancient philosophies. Our 5 stage process is focussed on achieving maximum change in the shortest amount of time possible.

Step #1: Evaluate

The first step in your Quality Mind journey is to become conscious of your mind's command of reality, and to expand that consciousness — a process that puts you into the flow of life, so that life flows to you! You no longer have to chase it, because chasing it is the slower alternative. Instead, as your intellect and consciousness embrace your intuition, you become a happier person: one who charges towards your highest excitement with enthusiasm, pleasure, and enjoyment.

Unfortunately, most people in the world today either forget, or don't know what their highest excitement is; instead getting locked into these self-protective rituals of behavior that keep their lives sheltered and small. They do their jobs without joy, engage in the same thoughts and behaviors day after day, and anesthetize themselves with empty pleasures, and often medication.

When this happens, they are fundamentally out of alignment with their TRUE NORTH and why they are here on this planet. They can't hear themselves — the Master of their own destiny, over their Child's mind keeping them sheltered and 'safe'. Being this out of sync with yourself can create anxiety, depression, illness or hardship in other areas of life, such as in your performance on the field, in the court, on the pitch or wherever your sport takes you.

Take anxiety, for example. Anxiety is rooted in fear, which has been an evolutionarily-useful feeling for the human species. But we're no longer wresting our very survival from the teeth of Mother Nature every day in the twenty-first century, and once you're a competent adult, fear has no place in your daily life. Yet anxiety disorders affect hundreds of millions worldwide.

Chronic anxiety fractures your concentration, can cause heart palpitations, extreme fatigue and high blood pressure, and that's just for starters. The body is led by the mind, and all the sports science in the world won't keep you injury-free if your head isn't in the right space and in the game.

In the world of elite sport, an athlete's body, from both a conditioning and training viewpoint, is already at 100%. They really can't get much more out of their bodies these days. Sports science is incredibly sophisticated and refined, but if you ask a sports scientist why so many athletes are getting injured, they can't tell you, nor can they accurately predict when athletes will crash.

I know it's because those athletes' minds aren't at 100%. They're worried about the last game, or what the media is saying, or something else that doesn't matter in the NOW. Quality Mind can stop that process. It will get your mind as fit as your body, and it will set you on the path to reaching the top of your game with consistent performance and zero injuries.

Activity #1: Life Scorecard Assessment

The first step of the Quality Mind process is to EVALUATE yourself mentally, emotionally and spiritually. This requires you to take an utterly honest and unflinching look at yourself. You need to really understand where you are to begin with, before you can go on and conquer. Benchmarking is a critical part of our process. We're not just giving you platitudes and hoping for change, we're actually analyzing you from a structured point of view so you can get back on a track to condition your mind and build the life you want.

Set aside 3 minutes and work through the questions on the QM website www.qualitymindglobal.com under GET YOUR FREE SPORTS PERFORMANCE SCORECARD TODAY. Don't think too hard about any of your responses either, just go with your *honest* gut feeling. Once you've accomplished this you will receive your own scorecard, and it's only 9 quick multiple choice questions that you need to answer.

If you don't have internet, here is an example of the Scorecard.

- On a scale of 1 to 10 (from least to most), please respond to the following statements...

We start with the *Body* section of the QM Wheel. For each aspect of the Body, score yourself by drawing along the line from 1 to 10:

#1. Sleeping Patterns

What's your quality and quantity of sleep like?

#2. Diet

Are you eating a nutritious diet and hydrating well?

#3. Physical Fitness

How physically fit are you?

For the most part, athletes will score highly in these three areas of the Body. After all, there's usually a whole sports organization behind them, dedicated to building and training their bodies to perfection.

Next we move on to the *Mind*. Again, score yourself on a scale from 1 to 10.

#4. Language

What is your inner language like? Are you beating yourself up or building yourself up mentally? From the minute you wake in the morning to putting your head on the pillow at night, how many hours of the day were you speaking highly of yourself?

#5. Now

How much of your day are you spending in the present moment, really conscious of what you're doing now, versus thinking about the past or the future?

#6. Letting Go

How quickly do you let go and forgive yourself and others? Do you stew on things and hold grudges? Or do you always forego resentment and forgive quickly?

Next, we're looking into the *Soul* — or that piece of yourself that you can call your Master mind, if you like. Score yourself from 1 to 10 by drawing along the corresponding line:

#7. Self-Love

How much do you truly love being you?

#8. Excitement

How excited are you about life? For what's coming? For what you have? Living each day like it's your last.

#9. Awareness

How aware do you feel of something bigger than yourself? How connected do you feel to your innate wisdom or higher mind?

Once you've finished rating yourself on these nine aspects in each of the three key areas, print off your Scorecard and file it as you will need it again soon!

This exercise may or may not have made you uncomfortable as you began confronting truths about your life and your mind that aren't necessarily what you'd like them to be. That's good — it means you're waking up and truly taking stock, and this will drive the change in you once we give you the tools to achieve a Quality Mind.

If you're a professional athlete, I recommend that you complete this self-assessment twice a week: after the game, and midweek. This will keep you aware of any potential issues, and help you focus on staying with the program and keeping your scorecard wheel full so that you can keep rolling through game after game.

In the off-season, make sure you're still checking in with yourself by filling out the QM Wheel on a bi-weekly basis.

Once you've completed your scorecard, it's very easy for you to visualize the areas of your life where work is required for you to become injury free and performing at your best consistently.

Please look at the Scorecard like looking down at an artery in your body — if your connected lines are tight to the center, then your energy and blood flow is restricted, and that's bad for your life. You've got to clean it out so the artery is wide open and flowing with ease. When you're in flow you're racing toward everything you've ever wanted and life flows to you — as opposed to you chasing life, which can often be futile. As you can see from the following graph, these 9 questions are all focussed on tapping in to the intelligence of the heart, which in turn will provide you with more energy in every aspect of your life.

When your language to self is always loving ♥, when you see appreciation and live as often as possible in the now ♥, when you consistently forgive yourself and others ♥, when you truly respect yourself with a sense of love for yourself ♥, when you are following your highest excitement as often as possible ♥, when you are aware and connecting to your innate intuition ♥ — you're more likely to sleep and eat far better as well as take much better care of your physical health.

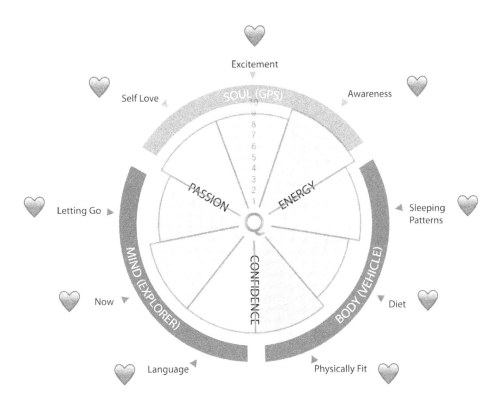

Take your free Sports Performance Scorecard today at www.qualitymindglobal.com

What Do You Seriously Want?

Once you have completed a clear evaluation, it's time to start thinking deeply about what you truly want from both your sports success and from your life, imagining that nothing is in your way whatsoever. This is something that you MUST get very, very clear on. If you're not dedicated to giving yourself an honest look, being straight about what your dreams are, and then fully committing to them, then there's nothing to work with. Here's a real life example:

Another athlete that I worked with during my time consulting for the Western Bulldogs FC was Easton Wood. He's an amazing talent, but he was always getting injured, and it was obvious to me that if things didn't turn around, he'd be on the chopping block. So I pulled him aside, and I said, "Easton, mate, you've got to be very careful here. You could be on your way out." He agreed, so I encouraged him to come and have a chat, but he was going to a mainstream psychologist at the time and he thought he was covered, despite his ongoing injuries. Finally, he conceded and he decided to come and see me. He was on his last legs, and had only played 5 games that season. For the first five years of his career, he was only averaging 9 games out of 22 per season.

In his first year with Quality Mind, we got him back to 18 games. He got himself in a great position and his confidence went up. In the second year, he said to me, "So what do I get this year?" I said, "What do you want?" He said "it would be nice to play all 22 games." I said "c'mon mate... that's short changing yourself... get serious...what do you really want? Do you want to be All Australian... win a club best and fairest? How about becoming a Premiership captain?"

His first response was, "That will never happen." "Well, then it won't and I won't work with you," was my immediate answer.

"Unless you want to go for the absolute gold medal, I won't work with you."

"I can't even imagine that," he said.

My reply was straightforward: "Well that's what we're here to do."

I directed him to visualize that success; I made him really feel it, and own it. I told him to bring it into the current moment and actually become it.

After some NLP and limiting belief busting I said, "Now tell me you're All-Australian."

He said, mumbling, "I'm All-Australian."

I said, "No, *tell me you're All-Australian*. I want to hear it." People were looking around in the office, but that didn't matter. They'd seen Jerry Maguire and, if not, they knew what we were there for.

"I'm All-Australian." Finally, after 4 or 5 attempts he was booming it out, and we shared a great laugh.

Bottom line: If You Can't See It, You Can't Create It

The body is subject to everything we're thinking and feeling because we are always creating. If there's excitement in life and a big carrot to chase, then there's enthusiasm towards where we're going, high levels of motivation and a surplus of energy. In 2015, Easton Wood won the Charles Sutton Medal (his club's best and fairest award) and became All-Australian. In 2016, he became the captain of the Western Bulldogs and won the premiership. His story is one of a remarkable turnaround, and he became recognized as one of the most elite players in the whole AFL competition. Easton's case study is featured in full further on.

What worked for Easton will work for you too, and we will cover this in more detail soon so that you too will have a super clear vision of what you're about to achieve (providing you follow my system and do the work, every day).

The Evaluation stage of our process is identifying and understanding the past, as well as how it continues to impact you today, so that we can get rid of it and get clear on where you are right now. To get you clearly focused on and excited for the future, and to drive up your excitement for what you can achieve.

Along the way, your use of the QM app will highlight for you and us when you're having a tough time, and when you're not. In fact, that's how the app was born. I'd be meeting with an athlete, and I'd ask how their week went. The response would come "Oh, Tuesday, I just was flat, exhausted, and Wednesday, I didn't recover well." But when I'd ask what happened or what they were thinking, the answer was always the same: "Oh, I don't remember." That drove the app's development, because that information was crucial.

With the app, I can go in on Tuesday, and I can see at 2:00pm they had a meeting with their coach who gave them a belting, or maybe they had a fight with their partner. It also gives me the opportunity to reach out in real time with a reminder to move into their Master's mind.

If someone doesn't want to truly evaluate themselves and start rebuilding their mind, we will know that rather quickly thanks to the Quality Mind app, because you have to use the app *every day* to change into the new you. The app is a powerful activation tool that helps create the next version of you, which involves expanding your consciousness and improving your health, happiness, and wealth. If you're not committed to the process, it will be very difficult to work with you. It's as simple as that. We won't work with anyone that is not 100% all in. To encourage this engagement, we've worked a variety of neurological motivators into the app from pleasure and reward, to self-improvement and self-direction, to pain and punishment.

One of the biggest motivators is a pain threshold, of course, since avoiding pain is a fundamental drive for all humans. If you don't use the app at least once every 48 hours, you get a strike. Once you get three strikes, you're locked out of the app for four weeks.

You'll also find a global leaderboard in the app that motivates you to keep on the right path and perhaps embrace a competitive camaraderie. Some people get quite inspired by that because they take pleasure in competition and are motivated by reward. They continually have fun with the rankings, and enjoy the banter that can build relationships with other people. Many people chat offline about it, and exchange playful taunts like, "I've got you! I'm at number five. I'll be number four soon." (You can list yourself under an alias on the leaderboard, too, for those wishing to go incognito.)

Case Study: Shaun Higgins

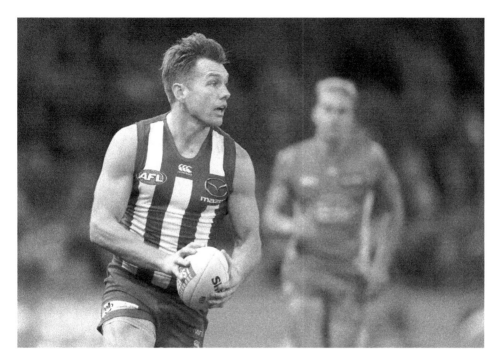

Shaun Higgins playing for the North Melbourne FC, AFL — Courtesy AFL Photos

Shaun Higgins plays for North Melbourne in the Australian Football League (AFL), where he has been awarded the Syd Barker Medal twice (as the best and fairest player of 2017 and 2018), as well as being named All-Australian in 2018 at 30 years old. A remarkable achievement for an AFL athlete.

Background: Plagued by Injury

Shaun fell in love with footy from an early age, inspired by his father's involvement in football. His dad, a builder, played reserves for Geelong FC before injuries got the better of him. This early exposure to football clubs ensured Shaun was a dedicated player in his junior years. In 2005, at the age of 18, he was recruited to the Western Bulldogs FC (AFL) on the back of his performance with the Geelong Falcons.

His professional debut came in 2006, but he suffered a season-ending injury just five games in with a dislocated elbow. While he proved himself as a critical and versatile performer over the years, the injuries kept mounting. During his nine-year stint with the Bulldogs, he faced shoulder surgery, a broken ankle, hamstring injuries, groin injuries, and that's not the worst of it. In 2013, three games into the season, Shaun suffered from a navicular fracture in his left foot, an injury notorious for resulting in diminished performance and chronic pain with a common recovery time in excess of one year.

Enter Quality Mind

Although he faced these physical challenges, Shaun demonstrated leadership qualities both on the field and in the locker room. He was promoted to the leadership group within the Western Bulldogs as early as 2009, and met Richard Maloney during the latter's time there as a leadership and culture coach with the club.

"I had spoken a little bit in 2012 to Richard about how I was feeling — I wasn't reaching my full potential, and there was something holding me back," Shaun said. "We got on really well and we chatted about the mental side of the game and the impact that it has for elite performance. If you got that right, then it really could unlock a lot inside you."

After he had surgery for his navicular fracture and faced fears that he might not play again, Shaun called Richard up to pursue a one-on-one mentorship in the early days of the Quality Mind program. Since he wasn't playing in 2013 due to the injury, he dove in headfirst to clean out his mind, connect with his deeper self and intuition, and become the player he knew he could be.

"In 2014, I got back and played the full year," Shaun said. He became a free agent at the end of that season and moved to the North Melbourne Football Club where he's been for the last five years. "It was really at North Melbourne where I reaped the rewards of the program. Continual challenges pop up, but Quality Mind gives you the awareness and the tools to be able to work through them."

"I played nine years at the Bulldogs where I was always seen as a player with potential, but never quite reached the heights that everyone expected. At North Melbourne, with the help of a lot of people and the work that I put in, I was able to become the player that I wanted to be. That resulted in 2017, 2018 winning the club Best and Fairest and, in 2018, being named All-Australian."

A Fundamental Shift in Thinking

"Early days for me, I thought that Quality Mind was just a quick fix. I thought that I had it. I'd do it and everything would be going really well, so I'd just drop off on what I was doing daily," Shaun shared. "Then a challenge would pop up and, before you knew it, I'd slipped back into the old patterns of thinking and behaving. That's the challenge: if you don't put in the work, then you can easily get off track again."

Using Shaun's Scorecard assessments from before winning the October 2018 Club Championship Award, and the All Australian Award (figure 1), then before his shoulder injury in June 2019 (figure 2), we can clearly see the positive effects of the Quality Mind program in action.

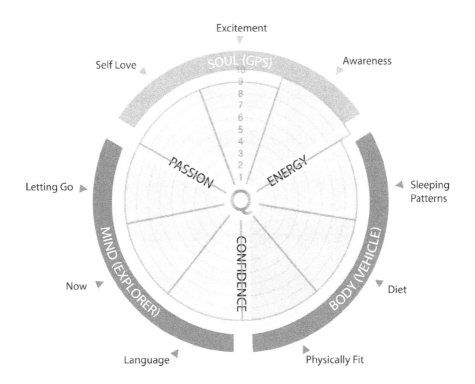

Figure 1. Shaun Higgins Scorecard reflecting his 2018 All-Australian & Club Best & Fairest seasons

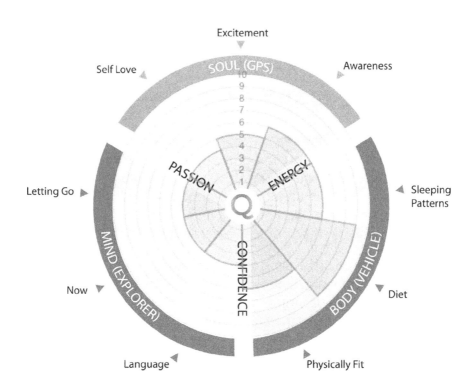

Figure 2. Shaun Higgins scorecard reflecting the shoulder injury sustained late 2019.

Figure 1 demonstrates where Shaun's head is at when things are going really well: "When you're in flow and things pop up, nothing sticks, and you're able to just flow through life knowing what you want to achieve, knowing it's there and then just letting it come to you."

"For me, when I slightly go off track and I know that I'm out of flow, which is what happened" (in figure 2), "you can see that I'm just trying to control the situation and control the outcome. I need to remember that will all take care of itself if I just remain in flow, remain excited, have a clear vision of what I want to do and what I want to achieve."

Shaun admitted that the biggest speed-bump leading up to the injury was that he was living in the future: "Being too focussed on the past, not being in the now, and feeling worried about my future resulted in a slight mishap and injury. Now, I'm able to step back and realize that, which helps make me even more accountable and aware of what's going on."

It's vital that an athlete controls all of the outside noise, like worry about the future, preoccupation with the last game, or addiction to the fame surrounding elite sports. When they achieve their Quality Mind, playing at the top of their game injury-free becomes effortless.

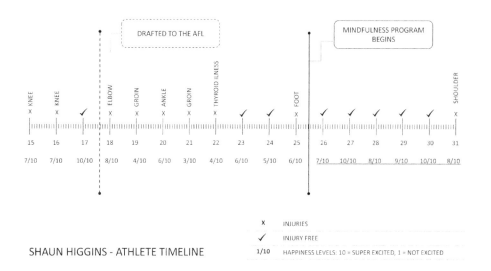

Shaun Higgins — Self assessed timeline graph reflecting his injuries and happiness levels.

As you can see from the timeline graph, once Shaun was drafted to the AFL at 18, he kept having injuries and breakdowns as his happiness in the game degraded. Upon joining the Quality Mind program at age 25, his career skyrocketed, and he recognizes that this emerged from his mindfulness program and the new mental foundations built on his Quality Mind journey. Shaun's track record is proof that these powerful techniques work — and are key to an athlete's mental foundation, made all the more effective if an athlete has the chance to have them instilled early in their career.

Energetic Mind; Energetic Life

When asked what achievements he's most proud of since starting the program, Shaun answered: "To get back and play consistent senior football at a really high level is one of the biggest achievements out of this and it definitely wouldn't have happened without the Quality Mind program. "

"The other achievements that I've created individually have been amazing as well — to win two Best and Fairests, I never thought when

I was injured that I would be able to do that. I always wanted to, but I could never close that gap between *wanting* to be that and being that."

Shaun has also found the Quality Mind app to be an invaluable part of the program. "The app enables me to have daily reminders to check in with myself constantly: make sure I'm present, make sure I'm living in the now, make sure my excitement levels are staying up and that I'm on track to reach the goals in my life."

In Closing — "Don't Force It."

"The Quality Mind transformation took place for me when I became aware of the importance of not forcing it, not controlling it, and not knowing how it *will* happen, just knowing that it will happen because I'm doing the work.

So does Shaun recommend the Quality Mind program to everyone?

"Yes, 100%. I say that because I use it in all areas of my life as well, not just sport, though that's the core part of my life at the moment. I use it, my wife uses it, my family members use it and they are all seeing amazing results. We all face challenges in our life, and it's great to have something that helps you deal with that — that also, on the flip side, takes you to whole new levels of energy and excitement and creating that you never thought were possible."

To access Shaun's full video testimonial please go to the Quality Mind Website: www.qualitymindglobal.com/success-stories/videos

Step #2: Retrain

Let's be clear on this one. We need to retrain our minds!

Throughout our childhood and adolescence we are not taught how to think, process and understand ourselves, or to grasp our unconscious and subconscious mind, which houses 95% of our mental challenges. It's not part of any school curriculum or parental handbook, and for most of us, our natural, untrained, default state is that of fear based thinking, which is not the basis for a Quality Mind.

The Journey of Three Stages

The Journey of Three Stages is a core concept of what you will learn, and it's the bare bones framework supporting the full Quality Mind process. It is the most fundamental key to your success on this journey of self-awareness and true power, and these three stages are:

1. Know thyself.
2. Accept thyself.
3. Become the conscious creator.

#1. Know thyself

The core objective of the first stage is to *know thyself* — which, from a basic perspective, means understanding what you're good at and what you're *not* good at. If you're about to take a hike up a mountain, you need to know that you don't have back issues or ankle problems. We went over this in Evaluate: understand your strengths, acknowledge what needs improvement and get clear on knowing who you are.

Getting to know yourself isn't always comfortable, and this journey will involve plenty of contrast, so don't worry if you feel like you're hitting more valleys of confusion than peaks of insight as you climb the mountain called 'Know Thyself.' Think of it this way: before you scale

Mt. Everest, you'll find yourself climbing and descending many smaller peaks. It's a process, and it's not a sprint.

Knowing thyself can be a tough journey, and it can take some time. If you're a young athlete still working through school or college, you might be fielding bullies or peer pressure, and still determining what kind of person you want to be. Or perhaps you're entering the workforce and you're not liking your job or the way you're reacting to that job or other people. Maybe you feel like you're always on the defensive with others, when you want to be open and generous. Or you feel constantly in others' shadows when you want to lead. This is the stage of honestly, truly knowing yourself. Who are you, and what do you want to become?

For example, when you first start playing a sport, you don't know the rules or how to strategize, and you might not perform very well. As you work on your game, you might face poor run times or performance stats, and you may have to deal with the pain and rejection of not making the team or winning the role you want. It hurts at the time, but it's all part of the journey to find out what you have to offer as an athlete as you build on your strengths and skills. Only when you know yourself can you then proceed to accept yourself and gain clarity on what you need to improve on.

#2. Accept thyself

The second stage is to *accept thyself*. When you enter this stage of the process, you'll notice that you're going down into fewer valleys and you're moving toward the top of the mountain more rapidly because of this self-acceptance. You've formed a good understanding of self-love and you've developed an appreciation of your own self-worth. This allows you to accept that you are perfectly imperfect, and that's not a paradox. You make mistakes but you get past those mistakes efficiently, learn from them and move on, without repeating them or allowing them to bog you down in anxiety or self-recrimination. You see it for what it is, growth. An opportunity to grow.

It's typical for most people to realize they've made a mistake and immediately attach a negative thought or emotion to that mistake. Mistakes often result in people feeling angry toward themselves and others. They might deny it was their own fault, and miss the lessons the mistakes offer them. These feelings of anger and disappointment can deepen into anxiety and depression, evolve into attitude or substance abuse problems, fracture a team's cohesion and more.

For the person who fully knows themselves and also accepts themselves, there's no emotion attached to the mistake. It happened: look at it objectively, understand what caused it and change your actions so it doesn't repeat without dwelling on it. You can do this with clear sight and positive energy when you're living from a space of self-acceptance.

Once you've achieved this (and our program shows you how) you've gone from knowing yourself to accepting yourself, which means you're ready to become the creator.

#3. Become the conscious creator

As you *become the conscious creator*, you have reached the understanding that we are all constantly creating. In this stage, you've reached the top of the mountain and you're fully in contact with your higher mind (more on the higher mind to come). You have yielded control to your greater purpose: where you're going, why you're going, and how you're getting there. This is what you need to realize: you are the creator within every moment of every day. You choose how to respond to every moment in your life, how to feel and how to act. When you fully take control of that, you create your own reality — one in which you move toward your highest excitement and your dreams with incredible energy, authenticity, and dedication.

We're Always Creating Anyway

Everyone on this planet has one thing in common: we are always creating in all ways, whether we like it or not, we don't get a choice! When someone says, "I'm not very creative," that's a belief they purchased for free from someone — a parent, a tv or a school teacher. They're not aware that they are always creating their life. (Obviously, there are different types of creativity: we're not talking creating art or coding an app or writing a book. We're talking about consciously creating your own reality, and it all starts and ends with a thought).

Metaphorically speaking, every moment of every day, we all have a paintbrush in our mind's hand, and consciously or unconsciously, we are painting pictures of our environment through feelings and thoughts. Most of us aren't even looking at the canvas, but we are still painting, and painting, and painting. Often we are blaming others for what is going on in our painting, and yet we are the one's holding the paintbrush. We are caught up in the past, or caught up in the future — and thus still painting poorly in the now.

What happens when it's time for you to actually have a look at the canvas (because reality is in your face for whatever reason) is you are confronted with a grey, blurry mess. There's no clarity, no defined picture, and no vibrant color. This realization that you've been painting all this time only to create a horrible situation for yourself can be an overwhelming blow. You haven't been consciously aware of what you've been creating, and so your life has been unwittingly heading down a staggeringly deep valley — in fact, you may be falling off a cliff!

Our goal is to get people to the stage where they're consciously creating: they've got the paintbrushes in their hand, they know what paints they're dipping in, from beautiful pinks and hopeful yellows, to calming blues and passionate reds, and so on. With their colors selected, they're focused entirely on their craft and their canvas. Throughout the day, they're completely aware of what they're thinking and what they're feeling, which are the real colors creating their painting. They are constantly building their future, excited by life, and arriving at the point where everything starts flowing to them.

When you're unconsciously creating and looking at your mess, you're always chasing life and it's got a fair head start. Once you get to the point where you're consciously creating, something amazing happens. You can evaluate your art, change the direction of your creation, and quickly make changes on the run to keep you on track. You're not emotionally enslaved to the outcome, but you know exactly where you're going, what you're doing, and what you want to achieve, all while remaining completely excited and full of clarity. When you complete your masterpiece, summiting the mountain and achieving your dream, the artwork is complete. It's beautiful; it's whatever you want it to be. It's your dream, and it's come to you effortlessly with no chasing required.

Once you reach the top of the mountain, there will always be another mountain for you to climb, should you choose to — that's life. However, you'll notice that the mountains become flatter. In other words, you get there quicker, and more easily, and it's not as harsh or as cold up at the top of the mountain. It's beautiful and euphoric, and the options available to you are boundless. You can continue to advance to the next mountain, but there won't be any valleys, as such. You'll just discover a higher understanding and a superior perspective on life.

During the Journey of Three Stages — especially when confronted with the creation of their own reality — people often push back because they don't want to know themselves. They're afraid to see themselves clearly, and they struggle with the concept of yielding control to their higher mind. Why? Because people are control freaks, and the majority of us are control freaks because we are out of control. When people have their nails bitten down because of to-do lists that contain 40+ items every day, they are probably feeling completely out of control. While we're out of control, we desperately want to control. It's a cyclical, habitual response rooted in anxiety, and it's just as useless. Have you ever tried to hold onto a handful of sand by squeezing your fist? You lose more sand than you keep. But when you relax your hand, the sand sits in your palm. The Quality Mind program helps you open your fist, and walk hand in hand with life.

These concepts are tough because most people don't know why we are here on this planet. If you don't know why you're here, if you're constantly seeking safety and certainty to control every minute of every day, then you're staring at the ground under your feet instead of the stars over the mountain. You're missing the great mystery of life. Why are we here? That's the question that underpins this whole program. It's the question that compelled me to start searching when I was 21 years old.

When I was going through school, I would have definitely been diagnosed with Attention Deficit Disorder (ADD), no question about it. They didn't have that box to tick at the time, however, so every one of my report cards said, "Has all the ability but is too easily distracted."

Throughout those years, what kept me happy was my sport: it gave me both an identity to hang my growing psyche on, and an outlet for the release of my anger. I was an angry kid. Even when going through two different schools, not connecting with the traditional academic methods of education, and challenging psychology at every opportunity, I was simply asking the big questions to gain certainty and clarity in my life. But there wasn't anyone to show me the way; I just kept coming up in contrast with my life. I was trying to get to the top of the mountain, but I didn't know where the top of the mountain was, or what it looked like.

All of that early contrast in my life was, quite simply, my higher mind pushing me to continue learning until I found my passion, which is this industry. I faced deep struggles to truly know myself and accept myself. I experienced depressive moments and high anxiety, but my intuition kept driving me through it all until I discovered my true purpose on life's journey.

Now I'm climbing mountains all the time, and it's really exciting for me to keep achieving these summits and to help others do the same.

We've clearly established that metaphorical mountains are a huge part of the Quality Mind program, and now it's time to break down your metaphorical mountaineer — who isn't metaphorical at all. There are three key parts of you that make up the mountain-climbing experience.

Vehicle / Explorer / Intuition

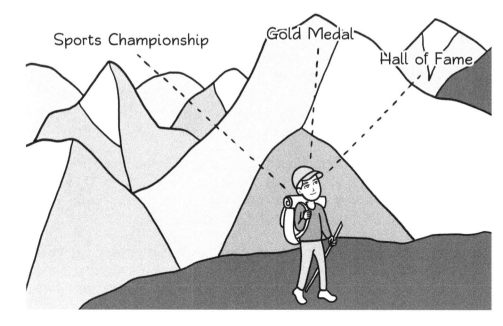

Everyone, throughout their lives, is climbing mountains. They're metaphorical, but they're still there, and each peak represents something that you want out of life. One peak may be becoming captain of the team, another peak may be winning a championship, a third peak may be scoring an endorsement deal. Whatever dreams you may have, there's a corresponding mountain peak to summit.

So if all of our dreams are at the top of each metaphorical mountain, then we obviously want to know the quickest way to the top of those mountain peaks!

So here it is. The quickest way to the top of the mountain peaks is to have 100% balance of these three key human components:

1. The *body / vehicle / physical* is the *modality* to get you to the top of the mountain.
2. The *mind / explorer / thinker* is the *hiker* who is wanting to climb the mountain.
3. The *soul / intuition / GPS* is your *innate* mind guiding you up the mountain.

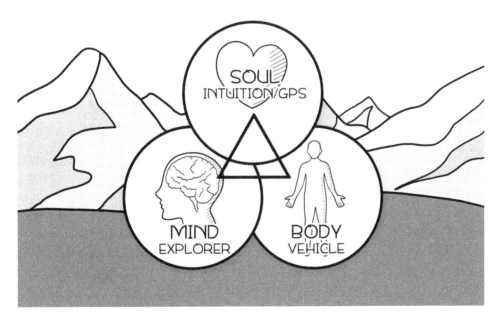

The *body / physical is the vehicle* so it needs to have the capability to climb the mountain.

Your *mind / explorer / thinker* is the decision-maker, who thinks it's responsible for getting you up the mountain.

The *soul / GPS or higher mind*, quite simply, is that part of you that's already been to the top of the mountain and knows how to get there, just like an experienced Sherpa. That Sherpa lives within you right now.

Understanding and aligning these three core elements will get you to the top of any mountain, and quickly. And remember this: whilst we may not know the exact reason why we are here on this planet, we do know we are on a journey to have new experiences and learn new things during our lives, and to express who we want to be along the way. True creators.

As we've discussed, the mind's job is to keep the body safe, and to preserve your human existence for evolutionary purposes. Your mind is constantly evaluating your surroundings and making sure everything is safe and in good order so that your body can push up and through to the top of the mountain. Our mind wants to be in charge, and we allow it to have all the power and all the control. That sounds okay in theory — except that without sufficient training, our minds are immature and stuck in default mode: ruling from fear, worrying about everything, preoccupied with the future, and obsessed by the past.

In reality, if we come right down to the mind's original coded purpose, it is simply designed to process the physical experience to keep you safe, and then to just silently go along for the ride. Your mind should allow you to walk into a room, look around, and say, "Yep, it's safe, it looks good here, no worries." Then it should get out of the way. But we've given it far too much authority and control, which gives it the weight to burden us with negativity.

You'll see many athletes so stuck in their minds that they're essentially letting a twelve year old pre-teen make their adult decisions. They are angry all the time, feeling like victims, and frustrated with always trying to be safe. It's a cyclical event, and once they start to realize that there are two key decision-makers here — not just the mind (which we will refer to from here on as your *Child's mind*), but the higher mind or soul (which we will refer to from here on as your *Master's mind*) — then we empower them through the Quality Mind toolkit to break the cycle, interrupt negative or unproductive thoughts, and replace them with thoughts at a higher vibration.

For reference throughout this book, we will refer to the *MIND* as the *CHILD* and the *GPS* as the *MASTER*.

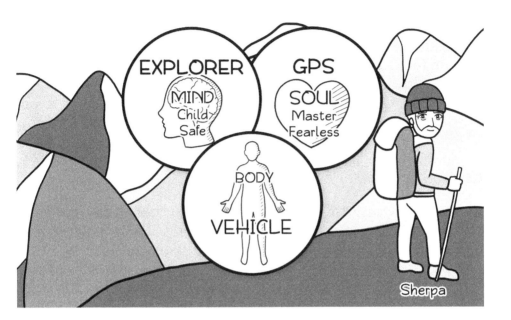

The Four A's

Your mental training to accomplish this level of control starts with embracing your intuition — that part of you that knows where you want to go and already knows how to get there — which we do through a process called "the four A's":

- *A*wareness
- *A*cceptance
- *A*cknowledge
- *A*llowance

I'll soon break these down individually, but essentially what you're trying to do is to recognize, acknowledge and connect to your intuition or innate wisdom on a consistent basis. By doing this successfully, you'll get to a zone where life flows to you as opposed to you always chasing life. Your intuition is like a GPS. If you imagine that your goal, or what you want to be, is a mountain peak, your intuition is that part of you that's already at the top of the mountain. It's calling down to you, "Just come this way and follow me. I'm already at the top of the mountain, you don't need to worry about the past, you don't need to worry about the future, just listen to me, and come this way."

If you are an athlete really excited by playing your sport and full of passion for your career — really feeling all of it deep in your heart — then you can accomplish anything. Anything! And that little voice in your head right now saying, "yeah, right, what the hell does he know?" is your Child standing in your own way. You're not looking at the mountaintop. You must embrace the awareness of your intuition, accept that it's there, acknowledge that it's about releasing control, then get out of the way to allow life to flow through you.

Anything you want in life can be accomplished, but because the untrained Child mind is in charge, and not just in charge, but a control freak and a dictator of your reality, it's going to show your reality through the perspective of a 12 to 13-year-old child, because again, it is programmed to keep you safe. Do you want to be mentored and led through life by a 12-year-old, consumed by selfishness and hobbled by the overwhelming obsession to keep safe? If the answer is yes, then you can stay in that reality, and we can't work with you. But if you want to move ahead, toward your dreams, and find life and abundance flowing to you, start with this truth: there are two key decision-makers inside of you.

The first is the higher mind, which we call your Master, and your Master is YOU. You just haven't been connected to your intuition because you haven't been able to hear it. You're not communicating with it. Once you start getting reconnected to yourself through your intuition, you will find yourself playing your sport, and living everyday life, with far more energy and enthusiasm. Your intuition is pure energy and pure intelligence, as opposed to your other key decision-maker.

This other mind is your Child mind, which is made up of emotions such as worry, fear and concern, all of which drain your energy. The Child mind is really a controller — it's power-hungry, impatient, and fearful. It's worried about the future and the past, it has low self-worth and it's moody. It's also very emotional, and when we are emotional, we lose energy. The Child mind is basically like a petulant child that's out of control!

The Master, or the higher mind, on the other hand, is a central intelligence — it is raw energy. Living in tune with your intuition means taking complete ownership of your every thought, sensation, action and decision. The Master is passionate, filled with purpose, excited, understanding and forgiving. And it's starting point is located in, around and behind your heart space.

Where the energy of your Child mind is rooted in the brain, your Master mind is rooted deep in your heart.

Once we reconnect you with your Master mind and you start getting in touch with your Master, you'll start seeing dramatic changes happening quickly. Let's look at an example of the average elite athlete's daily thoughts during the season:

Odds are, you are spending the majority of your time in your Child's mind, which means you're worrying about the game, reevaluating the game, rethinking the game, worrying over comments from the coaches, watching and listening to the media, getting involved in the media, obsessing over the media, listening to your teammates, worrying about the possibility of getting dropped, and more. Perhaps you didn't do a great execution of a kick, punt, tennis lob, whatever your sport is, and you repeat and replay that performance over and over in your mind obsessively. The Child is a control freak and it locks you into repetitive worry that tends to snowball.

This is when your Child may start to say via your subconscious, *"Alert, alert... listen, listen, this is way too much for you to handle right now and I'm concerned. You're stressed out of your mind, and you don't deserve this! I'm going to make a decision and I'm going to sit you out of the game for the next few weeks because you need a break and I want to keep you safe."*

This is when injuries and sickness occur, because the body is listening to the Child mind, and because everything is connected. It thinks it's protecting you.

If you're out of alignment, out of sync and not heading toward releasing all of this fear and worry, you're not connecting to your intuition. Your Master is always trying to help you, but if you're in this space then it can't help you because you're not able to tap in to it or hear it over the Child that has taken control. What happens next is you find yourself heading down the path of injury, illness, and / or inconsistent performance.

Let's flip this on its head. What happens when you come out of a game in full sync with your Master?

When you come out of a game and do your personal 100-Point Plan — which is in the programme — you recognize the strengths in what you did, you understand what you've learned, and you accept the facts of your performance. You don't get emotionally connected to it; instead, you clean it all down, move on from the past, and don't worry about the future. Forgiving yourself for any mistakes will keep your energy high, and as your energy remains high, you can freely look forward to the next game because you have released everything and you are continually living in your Master throughout the week. When you do that week-in and week-out, your energy goes through the roof. You vibrate with high energy and potential that is ready and waiting to become accomplishment.

Again, contrast this with living in your Child mind — when you worry about everything, your energy gets depleted. You start playing your sport with low energy, and that means you start making more skill errors. Over the course of time, your errors compound each other, and you may find yourself getting benched, removed from the team, or not chosen for the following week. All of a sudden, you're in a cycle again, and that cycle is a loop of negative feedback, which creates low self-worth.

This is the depressed level where I first connect with many of my athletes, because they get into that cycle and injuries start happening in the face of their low energy and low self-worth. Remember, the body is led by the mind. When your Child mind says things like, "this is far too stressful. I'm not sure if I'm good enough. I'd rather be surfing. I can't be bothered anymore. I'm tired of this. I'm out of my depth." — your body will create a reason for that break. You're always creating, and that means you're always creating your own reality. It doesn't matter what happens: it's what you *do* that matters.

We're teaching our athletes that when they live in their Master mind, they've got extreme levels of energy, as opposed to living in their Child's mind, with minimal levels of self-worth, energy, happiness, satisfaction, and success. I've never personally met a 12-year-old that's a multi-millionaire and has high levels of continued and sustained success.

Enter Awareness. This first stage of *The Four A's* is about understanding the characters of your Master and your Child, and being aware that your Child can never grow up. It is coded to keep you safe, and that is its primary and only role. The process is not about eliminating the Child; it's a key part of you and it has its use.

Embracing awareness is about understanding your two selves and recognising who is centre stage in all moments of your life. Awareness is the first and most critical step, because if you're aware that the Child has taken over, you can then take the necessary steps to bring your Master to the forefront. Then in time, once you are in full control of your Child, you'll find that they will merge.

The Master and Child need to be in perfect flow for the body and the mind to work together to maintain a healthy, harmonious, injury-free life. You need them both to flourish, but the Child must be controlled. You need to separate them first to understand their respective characters, strengths, and weaknesses, and to create awareness. By the age of 16, we know that we're reasonably safe, how to walk across the road, when people are possibly being dishonest, and what foods to eat etc. However, you still need your Child's mind with its preoccupation with safety, because if humanity didn't have that, we wouldn't be here — we would have taken too many risks. The Child is key for evolutionary purposes.

Your Child is usually like an actor on the stage: from the minute you wake up in the morning, you are in consultation with that actor, and it's a drama queen trying to capture your attention all day long.

We teach our athletes not to get abusive toward their Child; we just help them to start looking in a different direction. Initially, the Child will stomp its feet and say, "No, no, no. Do not look away. I'm in control here. What are you thinking? This is crazy. You're going to do a Quality Mind program? You're going to change direction? No chance. I'm in control, so don't look away."

This is where some people struggle: when you first start looking away, the Child on stage usually becomes more dramatic and demands more attention. But it's like any actor — if they're not getting paid, then they're not going to perform. Having said that, you still like to watch the act on stage, it's still fun to have a personality and uniqueness. We're not taking that away from anyone.

The bottom line is, when it comes to the bigger decisions in life, especially when you're a lead sportsperson, it's ludicrous to think you have time to spend in consultation with a 12 or 13-year-old. It's now time to speak to your ageless, intuitive Master mind that's ready to bring you all the accolades you want to achieve.

So in closing, Awareness is about understanding and recognising the characteristics of your two selves, so you can bring yourself back to your Master whenever the Child unnecessarily takes the stage.

Acceptance: This second stage is all about accepting that if you want to be the best in your competition, you have to start living that state of vibration in your Master every day. You have to begin visualising, imagining and knowing, taking vivid mental note of how this level of success feels.

I think, therefore I am. The laws of attraction. Like attracts like, etc. If you achieve this then your Master mind is already there, and the success will surely follow. You simply need to connect with your Master mind, because it can and will fast track you to where you want to go, providing you continually see it, feel it and believe it.

On the other hand, if you remain in your Child's mind, constantly questioning yourself, you'll be on the slow track, and you may never make it at all. You may achieve a certain measure of success, but it will not be sustainable and you will ultimately find yourself heading right back down to that familiar grey valley of mediocrity, frustration and potential injury.

Where you invest your energy dictates the focus of your life and the caliber of your performance. If you're in consultation with your Child's mind, your reality will only include childish outcomes, and if you're not in sync with your Master mind, you're not in alignment with your true purpose, thus creating unnecessary challenges and hardships. Once in sync, you will move out of the shadows and you will thrive and flourish in the sunlight.

Acknowledging is all about about appreciating and understanding that your Master is far more powerful than you could ever imagine or truly understand in this human existence. It's also about surrendering to the fact that we may never truly understand everything, and that's okay!

Your Master is connected to every element of the universe. It is the universe, and so are you. Everything is connected, and when we acknowledge this, we are truly in flow. *Acknowledging* is about embracing the knowledge that your dream is coming to you by being in flow with your Master (and by extension, your life). This step further builds the foundation under acceptance, because you're acknowledging that you are receiving and moving towards your goal. Nothing can stop you because your higher mind is already there.

Allowance: This is the final stage in *The Four A's*, and it's simply about allowing your Master through. The quickest way to embrace your Master is by acting it, and we do this by making a considered choice about virtually everything in our day to day lives. Consider how your Master would act, feel or be in any given situation, and choose that higher path. Consider what would my Master choose, or how would my Master react to this? It's about making thoughtful and conscious decisions about how you think, how you feel, how you relate, how you invest your time and who you want to be. With *Allowance*, it's easy to identify who's in charge and to make a better choice if your Child is at the helm. Where your Child may choose anger, guilt, bitterness or blame, your Master will choose empathy, kindness and understanding.

Allowance is about taking that final leap, releasing control and getting excited by your everyday existence, without worrying about the future, or about when or how it comes. It's about living in the now and allowing yourself to know and trust that you're on track. You're no longer playing your sport from a place of fear, worry or concern. You're not trying to control your contracts, you're not trying to control the coach's outcome, you're not trying to control anything more than what you can control: your own performance. You are simply living moment by moment with clear, exciting dreams that you are passionate about and you are determined to achieve.

Basically, if you're fully present and plugged in, what you're after will come to you if it's on your path, assuming you have the physical attributes and the training memory to perform at the highest level. It is like putting your hands in the air and saying, "I'm allowing this to take place. I know that I'm on track. I'm going to allow my higher mind through, and I'm going to stay excited, and watch my thinking, not go into the future, not sit in the past, and consistently keep my thinking in that place of "I love life, I'm safe. I love dominating on the field."

By following these four As, you'll find that your Child's mind can't control you anymore, because your Master has taken over and you keep it that way by staying in that present moment. Remember this, because it's important: the more you're in the past and the more you're in the future, the less energy you have and the more you lose. Dream and have a plan for the future by all means, but don't hold onto that plan so tightly as you will only focus on your hand, and not the bigger picture. The more you're in the present moment, engaged in and seeing perfection in the present moment, the more perfection you can create. You're giving and receiving, and what you put out is what you get back. This is a universal law.

Acknowledge that you are at the top of the mountain and that you've already reached your goal. It's now just got to be played out through feeling it, and becoming it, as a start. It's like you've already written the script of what you want, and now you must simply play out that role. Unfortunately, what often happens is that people go on stage and they think they've lost the script. Then they experience uncertainty, doubt and fear. Don't let that happen! Acknowledge that you are on stage with your script, and allow everything to proceed as its been scripted without overthinking. In a nutshell, get out of your own way! Stay excited for your future, but don't grab at control over when or how it comes. Finally, keep your Child off the stage whilst you learn to balance the both, and you will be guided toward your dreams.

Practice Makes Perfect

The innate Master is a muscle that I am asking you to exercise and use constantly, and one of the easiest and most effective ways in which to do this is by consciously trusting your first intuitive thought. Honor the fact that your first intuitive thought is often the most powerful level of communication your higher mind has with you.

For example: When you are walking down the street and you see a beggar your first intuitive thought is empathy. "I want to help." It comes from the heart (which is where the higher mind is centred).

Then, almost instantly your Child mind (who thinks it's in charge) will take over and say practical things like, I don't want to encourage begging, or they'll just spend it on alcohol or cigarettes or they should get a job, and consequently you are more likely to just walk on by. Sound familiar?

Learn to recognize intuitive thought. Learn to hold it longer if you can, and stop and analyze what it was if you can, because you must take the conceptual intuitive part of your body, which is the innate Master, and work with it in unison with the intellectual brain. In order to do that, you've got to embed it, by practicing the four A's and making it a habit. You've got to see it for what it is, and understand it. It's not easy at first, but it gets easier as soon as you open yourself to the four A's.

You can use intuitive thought everywhere. Many of us already do in the guise of the parking angel! You involve this seeming outside source to find you a parking spot because you can't see the whole car park, and you trust it. And you'll turn left, and you'll turn right until this space opens up. You feel that you have used an energy that is beyond yourself, which you then call the parking angel, but you also understand at the intuitive level do you not? That you just used your own intuition. This is a fun example of exercising your Master, but an example nonetheless.

You can talk to and exercise your Master in many interesting ways, and these stretch far beyond intuitive thought. You can even muscle test it, and one highly effective way to do this is via Kinesiology. Kinesiology is used in the complementary health and natural medicine field, and it is defined primarily as the use of muscle testing to identify imbalances in the body's structural, chemical, emotional or other energy in order to establish the body's priority healing needs and evaluate energy changes

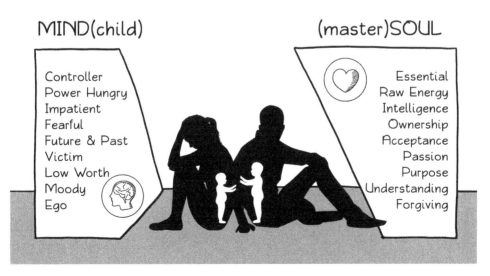

Diving deeper into understanding the personality of the Child mind and the Master mind.

brought about by a broad spectrum of both manual and non-manual therapeutic procedures. Google it to find out more. It really works!

Your Master is also responsible for the chills of discernment or inspiration. Right now you may be feeling the fact that this is true. When you get chills or goose bumps, that's so often your Master jumping up and down and saying, "Listen, listen, listen, listen." So make sure you do!

Delving into Thought Shopping

The most frequently used activity in our Quality Mind process (and app) is also the one that teaches you our key method for aligning with your Master mind. It will inspire you to live within your heart centre, moment by moment and day by day. It's called 'Thought Shopping.'

Consider: what sort of thoughts would your Master mind have? What sort of power statements would your Sherpa be screaming at you from the top of the mountain? What would those provocative comments and belief statements be? Those statements might be:

- Life is amazing; love the journey.
- You're on track.
- You are fearless and always know what to do next.
- You are safe; there's no better time to take risks.
- You are financially free, because I've already got all the money you need up here.

If you're in an executive business role, you might hear

- "you are a global thought leader."

As an athlete, it might be

- "you are an elite athlete,"
- "you're the best in the competition,"
- "you are All-American/All-Australian,"
- "you're a big game player and true leader,"
- "you play your best under pressure," and
- "you dominate every game."

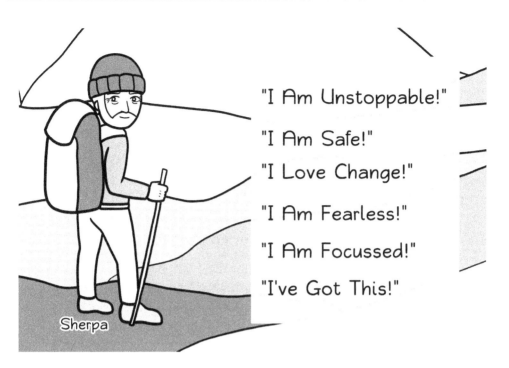

We're using the word *you* here, but we want them to turn it into *I am*. "I do this. I am fearless. I am focused. I am safe. I am unstoppable." The deliberate act of creating these power statements, organizing them, and using them to displace our old patterns of thought is critical to the Quality Mind process. Remember, we experience an average of 70,000 thoughts a day, and most of those are from our Child's mind. So, how many times do you think you need to go Thought Shopping each day so that you can use these powerful thoughts from your Master's mind to recode your brain and reroute your neurons? The answer is as many times as possible.

Generally, there are two parts to Thought Shopping. The first part is self-medicating — it's breaking away from the negative thought with a counter-thought that asserts "I'm okay," "I'm safe," or "I'm feeling good." This helps you quickly boost yourself out of the Child's mind so that you're sitting in your Master's mind.

What's important is embodying the new thought. We're not just retraining the brain and mind, but also the body. You must act out the statement, like it's already happened. For example, if you're focusing on feeling safe, you must go to that place of feeling safe: once your Master mind tells you, "you're safe, you're safe...I'm safe..." it's crucial to internalize that statement. Act it, Feel it, Become it.

The Child mind won't like this to start with. It will challenge it because it tries to use its own logic — which is skewed. But logically, you are safe in that given moment. Bring that inside of you and then experience that feeling of being safe. Convince yourself that you're safe. Close your eyes and stay in that position for 10 to 20 seconds. Really feel what that feels like in your heart space.

For a pro athlete, another example might be, "I've had my best game ever." They can sit in what it feels like to be best for those 10 to 20 seconds. Odds are, they've actually been there in the past, multiple times, so they can recall the feeling of being the best on the field. They can take that memory and bring the feeling into their body in the present.

The more you Thought Shop and deliberately change your thoughts and feelings throughout the day, the more you're changing the vibration of your body, which changes your energetic frequency outside of your body. Again, at the start you need to create multiple power statements that you think a Master would say, then act upon what you create and keep repeating it in yourself: "I am unstoppable. I am unstoppable. I am best on the field." See it, feel it and act it. Move through life like you're already at the top of your mountain. Walk in everyday life feeling your future self, act as your future successful self and very soon you will become it. Again, what you put out, is what you get back.

Thought Shopping empowers you to deliberately stop the onslaught of childish, negative thoughts that flow through your mind and then into your body. We're arresting the momentum of your old way of thinking. For example, if you've had a bad game and come off the field, then your Child's mind most likely kicks into gear and says, "You weren't good enough. You're going to get dropped from the team. Your contract's gone." These thoughts can and do snowball and can last for hours, days, weeks and months.

This is why it's so important to teach our athletes that you've got to watch the momentum in everything you're thinking all day long until it becomes your new normal. Quite simply, we want to re-code our minds so that the Master is now on stage, not the Child. That is what it means to be completely clear and aligned in your thinking and your feeling.

It's like stopping a driverless car at the top of the hill before it careers downward in an undirected rampage. If you wait until momentum has taken hold and the car's almost down the hill before jumping in front of it, you're not going to stop the car. You're going to get wiped out, run over and injured. You've got to interrupt the momentum early on, and this is true in everyday life, as well as in the high pressure lives of elite athletes.

Retrain your mind and body: stop the momentum of the Child's mind, connect with your Master's mind, and become the version of you who is the best in the competition, or the leader of the team, or the strongest in a certain position. If you can't get out of the feeling in your body and into your future self, you can still bring an old memory back in that reminds you what it feels like to be best on the field. You should stay there, remember that time, own that feeling of success, walk that, act it out and become that for as long as possible. This disrupts the old patterns and removes the old thought process, leaving your body free to rise to a higher level of energy.

The second part of Thought Shopping is becoming the creator, just as in the Journey of Three Stages. We've put strategies in place to remove that negative, low vibration thinking, and we've brought in the new power statements from your Sherpa at the top of the mountain. So you've self-medicated, and now it's time to move into the future and create what you want.

"I am the best player in the competition," even if you're not there yet. You will be; your Sherpa already is.

"I am a Superbowl player." You're moving into the future, embodying how it feels to be that success and live your dream. You're manifesting it in the now.

The floodgates open at this point, with our clients realizing that they can create anything they want, and that the sky's the limit. You're flooded with high energy, and we want to direct that into the positive by really acting out your Master's mind. Remember, the intuitive Master mind represents your best self, and this process is all about getting back to who you really are, while simultaneously cleaning out what you've become — which is probably 70,000 thoughts of mostly worry, concern and limiting beliefs.

Activity #2: Dreams and Fears

To get started with Thought Shopping, you must first confront some of the fears and limiting beliefs we all have. Take the next five to ten minutes, and consider this question: "What is it that is holding me back? What fearful discussions am I frequently having with myself?"

You can apply this to any area of your life. What is holding you back from being the best defensive linebacker, the best ruck, the best point guard? What is holding you back from reaching your financial goals? What is holding you back from becoming the captain of your team? What is holding you back from maintaining a healthy romantic relationship?

Your reasons are incredibly personal to you, of course, but I can identify a few broad answers that we've heard often from our clients:

- I'm not good enough.
- I'm not smart enough.
- I'm not making enough money.
- I don't have enough time.
- I don't deserve to be successful.
- I'm afraid of what success will mean.
- I'm not healthy enough; I keep getting hurt.
- I don't have the support I need.

Each of these statements immediately puts you in a low vibration, leaving you moving through a world of humiliation, regret, anxiety, and self-sabotage. They're useless and negative, and even if they seem to be true, they're not true. So it's time to select your first power statements to use in thought shopping.

Think about those things you wrote down, and the stories you're telling yourself about what's holding you back. Then turn that thought upside down: what is the exact opposite of your thought?

"I'm not good enough" becomes "I am unbelievably amazing" or "I'm the best damn running back in the league" or "I am a master at my sport."

"I'm not making enough money" becomes "I have all the money that I need" or "Money comes to me effortlessly and easily" or "I am an elite athlete and more money is on its way, baby!"

"I'm afraid of what success might mean" becomes "I am super excited by success and I can't wait to see what new opportunities it brings."

"I'm not healthy enough" becomes "I have a perfectly conditioned body that gets stronger every moment of every day."

"I don't have the support I need" becomes "I have a world leading team around me."

Whatever the opposite statement is, write it down in the language that is most powerful for you and your life. These statements should make you sit up straighter, feel pumped and get goosebumps. These are your "hell yeah!" mantras that are meant to elevate your vibrational state, and if you're not feeling that energy shift when you focus on your statement, you haven't made it powerful enough yet.

Put some music on and spend about twenty minutes brainstorming these first thought shops. Aim to come up with at least ten powerful statements that stop your negative 'Child' thoughts in their tracks and shoot you upward into a higher vibration and energy.

Make sure these statements all start with "I" and are in current tense — they should look like "I have…," "I am…," and "I know…." If you have any that suggest the future or obligation, discard those. Do not use "I need to…," "I want…," "I'll try…," and similar statements.

Once you've got your top ten final power statements, add them to your app. Open the Quality Mind app on your smartphone, and navigate to the Thought Shopping tab. Follow the directions on screen to enter your thought shops one at a time. You can add or remove these power statements at any time, keeping your thought shops relevant and vibrant for you. Whenever one just doesn't pack the same punch anymore, you can brainstorm another and evolve your list.

Practice Thought Shopping as often as you can each day, and especially when you recognize that you're in your Child's mind, being pummeled by limiting beliefs, or sliding into negative thought patterns. Simply open your app to the Thought Shopping tab, identify how you're feeling, and *why* you're feeling that way and assess your thoughts. Then select a thought shop from your list of your new power statements, and repeat it to yourself ten times — out loud, in your head, whatever works — until you *deeply* and *fully feel* your power statement in your body and in your heart. With your energy shifted and your vibration levels back up, you can return to your day knowing that you're rewiring your brain into a Quality Mind.

The Six Stages of Mindful Alignment

Before we move on to the next step in the Quality Mind framework, it's important for you to clearly understand how the body is led by the mind, and how being out of alignment with your Master mind and your highest excitement is the quickest way to mental hardship, physical injuries, and other ailments. This is easily seen in the Six Stages of Alignment as we walk from a thought to a sensation farther along a downward spiral, away from our true north.

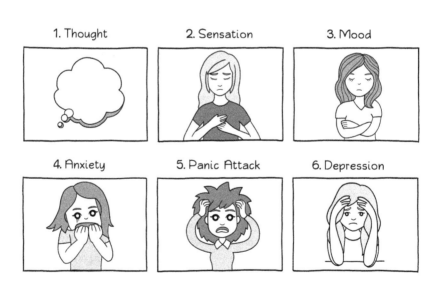

The Quality Mind Six Stages of Mindful Alignment

Stage One — The Thought

A thought goes through our heads at a million miles an hour, and we're not even aware of most of them. As you have already read, we have about 70,000 thoughts a day. Upwards of 90% of those thoughts are from the day before, which means most of our brains are on constant repeat. And a belief is merely a thought repeated enough times that it becomes a firm belief.

So, a thought that's well out of alignment with our Master mind comes in, usually quickly enough that we can't spot it. Sometimes, we may even be hiding these negative thoughts from ourselves, and if it's a thought that isn't working for your benefit like 'I'm not good enough,' you're going to find that you feel a low vibrational 'sensation' in your body.

Stage Two — Sensation

Depending on the thought or even before the thought if the body is triggered, you may feel a physical sensation in your chest, throat, head, neck, or in any part of the body. It's a sensation that is telling you, quite simply, that you're off track. When you can't track the 'Child' thought quickly enough, the sensation is your next warning light, signaling, "Alert, alert, alert! We've got the wrong thought going on here." Most people become so used to getting that sensation and they don't know where it's coming from, but it's coming from the thought.

For example, an athlete might have a concerned thought because they're worried about the game on the weekend, and that then manifests as stomach upset or gastric distress.

The body is always being triggered because we're a sponge of past experiences. These thoughts come in on the back of a range of stimuli, from game day footage from a previous season to the smell of a past partners' perfume or cologne to a certain song playing. Future worries are always nearby for most of us as well. So the sensation comes in and you feel it in your head, gut, heart, throat or anywhere in the upper body.

If you randomly find yourself taking a quick deep breath or hunching your shoulders or fisting your hands, these sensations are the clue or trigger that you are off track and you're in your Child, and if you don't take note of it and address it in its tracks, you're on the way to stage three.

Stage Three — Mood

Now you've gotten into a mood: as in moody, negative, and unpleasant. Your personality is your personal reality, meaning it's made up of your thoughts and feelings. When you've got inconsistent thoughts leading to negative sensations, you're left with an unhappy personality that's taking you nowhere fast. For example, you wake up one morning and get out of bed in a bad mood — because you're not a morning person, or because of an argument you had the previous night, or because of your poor diet. Maybe you're worried about your finances or a mistake you have made in last week's game. Whatever the reason, once the sensation is in your body and you're in a mood, it's easy for the downward spiral to continue. If it continues to stay there it builds momentum, which means the driverless car is now well and truly rolling down the hill.

Stage Four — Anxiety

Once this sensation gets momentum and the mood becomes a pattern — or even a routine — over time you're now entering into anxiety. This is when people start chewing their nails all the time, can't focus, are super sensitive to their outer world or wind up on medication. This pattern is now ingrained in their mind and body, a superhighway for their neurons in the brain to fire and wire. Anxiety becomes their reality, and this can then lead to panic attacks.

Stage Five — Panic Attacks

A panic attack is the most overwhelming sensation of all the sensations. The thought drops into your mind, manifests as a sensation in your body, which becomes a mood, then burrows in to become anxiety. Stage five is the panic attack because it is repeating at out of control rates, and it is all so overwhelming. The body is now completely consumed by an overload that can cause heart palpitations, shortness of breath, feelings of dizziness and more. Even worse, this stage comes with triggers that can bypass previous stages and throw you right back into stage five in the future. For example, a panic attack could get triggered in the workplace when an athlete has a profoundly unpleasant interaction with a coach or manager. Now, they can be triggered every time that person shows up to a meeting, since the body remembers the trauma of the previous experience, which leads us to the next stage.

Stage Six — Depression

Depression is the final stage of being well and truly out of alignment with your true north and highest excitement and living in the NOW. Its arrival can both be caused by and result in not wanting to go to work. Perhaps you are worried about future panic attacks, or maybe you didn't have any panic attacks, and moved from anxiety straight into depression. Everyone is different, but usually the sequence follows the series of stages I've laid out here.

The most critical element here is to understand this: when you stop the thought, you stop the sensation. You kill off this entire process if you can nip it in the bud in the first two stages and repeat and repeat and repeat until you re-code yourself. This understanding is the key to Thought Shopping, one of your primary tools in Retraining on our Quality Mind journey.

Four Universal Laws for Mindfulness

Every thought creates, and thoughts are powerful forces. They shape your understanding of reality, and they are responsible for the full shape of your life. What most people don't know is that this framework is governed by four universal laws that you must understand to command.

The Universal Law of Control

You are in full control of every thought you have. Many people will blame others for the way that they're thinking and might say, "You made me think that," or "you made me feel that." This is rubbish. It's on them. They're being reactionary and are out of control.

Think about what you want, not what you don't want. You may think that our thoughts are beyond our control, but that is never the case. We always choose our thoughts — every moment of every day. And our thoughts always have an effect — there are no neutral thoughts.

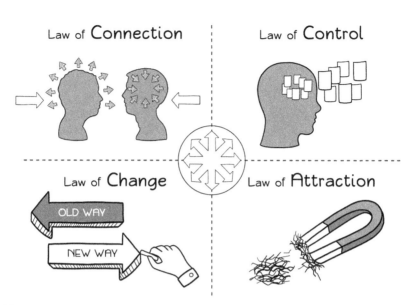

The 4 Laws

The Law of Change

Now that you know that you are in full control of your thoughts, you can appreciate the second law. The Law of Change states that you have a universal right to change every thought. You are in absolute full control, and you can change any thought at any time. Most people just don't know how to — or they don't want to, because they're loving the emotional drama that they're in. They're caught up in a cyclical, downward spiral of self-damaging thought processes; and they don't want to change, because they don't want to take ownership or responsibility.

People who suffer with anxiety will often blame their external world for this, when in fact it's quite the opposite. They choose to believe and accept that certain people or situations make them anxious, as though it can't be changed — when in fact nothing in your outer world can evoke your anxiety unless you create it and encourage it internally. For instance, why is it that when you see a certain person you feel anxious, whereas when you see someone else you feel peace and relief? The person has not caused your feelings — it's an experience or a memory that is flooding back, and in the past you gave that experience a label. It's all you, and it's a choice. *Everything is neutral until you give it meaning.* When you bring this powerful statement in to your daily life, it alone will evoke great change in you. It really is that powerful!

The Law of Connection

If you can conquer this law, you're on your way to being the full master of your mind. The Law of Connection states that there is an inner world and an outer world. Everything within us and everything behind our eyes comprises our literal inner world. Everything outside of our eyes is the outer world.

These worlds may be separate, but they are also connected. Your outer world is a reflection of your inner world. If your inner world is out of control, you're going to find that your outer world is out of control. When you find people trying to control everything in their lives, you can bet their inner world is out of control. They try to control people and every circumstance. They try to force their way on the world and others, and in the process, they upset people and they live out of flow.

If you look at all of the best winning sports teams, usually their on-field success is a reflection of their off-field success. There is good management, good administration, good structures, and good flow in place. The same thing happens off the field, which means they get that success on the field. It flows.

The Law of Attraction

Whatever's happening in your inner world, whether positive or negative, attracts its match in your outer world. If you're consistently full of fear, worry, concern and doubt, then you're only going to attract more of that in your life because it's what you're creating. Everyone reading this book right now needs to understand, that according to the Law of Attraction, their current environment has been completely created by themselves.

And if you're unhappy with your current environment, then you've got to start separating yourself from your outer world, and we'll show you how to do that in the Cleaning step of the Quality Mind process. You'll start to see that when your inner world is cleaned out, your outer world cleans down, and then the Law of Attraction works for you in the way that you want. You attract what you're putting out — and where your focus goes, your energy flows.

How Are You Vibing?

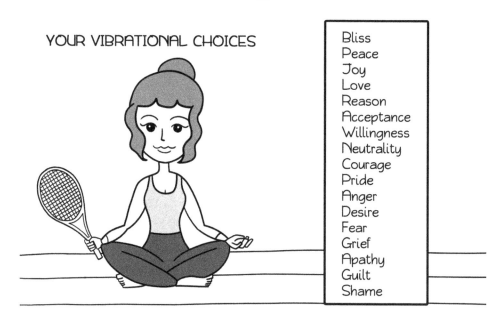

Vibrational Levels

You may have noticed that I frequently refer to your vibrational levels and the need to keep them at a high level. Learning how to raise your vibrational frequency is the single most important thing you can do to improve your life. By learning to raise your vibrational frequency, you will be able to create the biggest possible impact you can have on yourself and the planet as a whole. This shift is so powerful that it will change everything about you and the people you come into contact with. It is the foundation of this shift that will allow you to go out into the world and do great things if that is what you want and are destined to do.

All vibrations operate at high and low frequencies within us and around us. If your vibration is low, it will be evident. It's simply a matter of bringing awareness to your situation and then working on rectifying it, and it's another reason why the QM App was built. Perhaps you've never thought about your frequency before, but it impacts every aspect of your life. You create your own reality, and like attracts like.

Similar to radio waves that are heard but remain unseen, your vibrational frequency emanates from your cumulative thoughts, emotions, and consciousness and is continually being broadcast out into the world.

Here are 5 simple ways to quickly raise your vibration.

#1. Your Thoughts & Words

The power of sound is conditioning your mind to constantly experience what you speak. The words you speak to others, or to yourself, can actually be weakening your vibration and causing you to feel bad. Your words guide your mind and body towards the experiences you want to have. For example, choosing not to say anything negative for 24 hours will help you become more conscious of the things you say to yourself and to others. This is a wonderful challenge that you can do by yourself or with someone else. A lot of times we don't even realize how many negative things we say. Always keep the power of your words in mind. Vibration is influenced by thought, so just imagine how you can positively influence vibration with positive intentions. During your 24 hours, start saying more kind things to yourself and to others. Use your words to empower yourself, affirm exactly what you want to experience, change the words you speak to yourself and to others, and you will raise your vibration.

#2. Meditation & Relaxation

There are hundreds of meditations available to you on the app, and if sitting still is not your preference, we also offer powerful walking meditations that evoke an even greater effect.

The practice of meditation permanently strengthens the most evolved portion of the human brain, the frontal lobe, which is linked to increased abstract thought, cognitive reasoning, creativity and positivity. It also triggers the brain to release naturally occurring neurotransmitters including dopamine, oxytocin and endorphins, which are linked to different aspects of happiness — from simple pleasure to a deep sense of calm. Regardless of your religious orientation, or which method you choose to use to meditate, even five minutes a day can help you clear the mind, confront and minimize negative, conscious and unconscious thinking patterns and connect to the divine space within that transcends thoughts, feelings and circumstances. Over time, this practice will raise your energetic frequency and contribute to a happier, more uplifted experience of yourself, others and the world at large. This also helps you to raise your level of vibration.

#3. Gratitude & Appreciation

Taking a few minutes every day to wake up with gratitude will immediately raise your vibration and allow for more miracles in your life. Gratitude is one of the highest vibrations we can feel along with love, freedom, and empowerment. Starting your day with thoughts of gratitude can set the tone for the day. What are your first thoughts when you awaken? Make an effort to consciously start your day with gratitude, love, and peace. The energy of gratitude can help change your mood from a sour one to a blissful one. There is so much to be grateful for, and when we take even one minute out of our day to express gratitude, we are giving our soul a warm boost of love and focus. What are you grateful for? Making a gratitude list shifts your vibrations from focusing on what you don't have to what is already abundant in your life. There is more to be grateful for than you could possibly imagine. When you raise your vibration with gratitude, the universe responds.

#4. Body Nourishment

Besides positive thinking, the fastest way to increase your vibration is consuming foods and liquids that are filled with vital energy. Some foods vibrate at high frequencies and some at lower frequencies. Most importantly, pay attention to how eating certain foods make your body feel. You've heard the saying that 'you are what you eat.' Just remember this: every time you eat any kind of food, you're absorbing its energy into your body. The quality of that energy has a direct impact on the quality of your health and vibration level. Energy is the core substance of everything in the universe. Without energy, there would be no life. Understanding how energy frequency works is important for your wellbeing. When your energy isn't vibrating correctly, you are more vulnerable to illness, negative thinking and depression. Plants are filled with vital energy from the sun, which your body naturally understands. The more you consume high vibrating energy foods (and water of course), the more positive, energized, and vital you'll feel, ultimately raising your vibration.

#5. Audio Frequency

Since music is a type of frequency, you can easily raise your vibration by listening to music that feels good. It's like a vibration raising hack because it takes hardly any effort on your part to sit and enjoy a nice tune. Try it now! Sound and vibration play a fundamental role in everything. Every object has a natural rate of vibration. In fact, the human body is a symphony of sound. Every organ, every muscle, every system, every bone, every cell, no matter what size, they are all in a state of vibration. Everything that vibrates does so at a certain rate. This rate is known as its frequency. You can use the proper audio frequencies to positively alter your brainwave frequencies and produce specific desired results.

Solfeggio frequencies make up the ancient 6-tone scale thought to have been used in sacred music. Each Solfeggio tone is comprised of a frequency required to balance your energy and keep your body, mind and spirit in perfect harmony.

The main six Solfeggio frequencies are:

- *396 Hz* — Liberating Guilt and Fear
- *417 Hz* — Undoing Situations and Facilitating Change
- *528 Hz* — Transformation and Miracles (DNA Repair)
- *639 Hz* — Connecting/Relationships
- *741 Hz* — Expression/Solutions
- *852 Hz* — Returning to Spiritual Order

As you meditate along with this type of music, you will let go all of the negative feelings inside your heart and then watch it fill with love and positivity, giving you a higher vibration.

Again, the QM App has been built to help you maintain high vibrations and offers multiple tracks to suit your mood, time and outcomes. At the end of the day, what you put out is what you get back. That's also a non-negotiable universal law.

Tune yourself back to the perfect vibration

Albert Einstein stated: "Concerning matter, we have been all wrong. What we have called matter is energy, whose vibration has been so lowered as to be perceptible to the senses. There is no matter." All matter beings vibrate at specific rates and everything has its own melody. The musical nature of nuclear matter from atoms to galaxies is now finally being recognized by science.

That is why these frequencies are so powerful. They can literally bring you back to the original tones of the heavenly spheres and put your body into a balanced resonance. Just play the music!

Activity #3: Designing the New You (Part 1)

Athletes already know the power of visualization. It's been a popular practice in sport for decades, with athletes mentally rehearsing play strategies and performances before enacting them. It should come as no surprise that visualization also plays a large part in being the creator and consciously creating the life that you want.

Many people simply don't know what they want in life, so this activity is about defining what you want and building a collage of the places, people, concepts, and things that surround your future self. It's about visualizing your dreams as reality, and bringing that energy into your every day life.

For this exercise, we're starting with visualizing your goals in Lifestyle, Relationships, and Health. We've put together a series of questions for you to answer; you can do this in a few sessions, or in one big session, it's up to you. Simply take some time to go through the questions and answer them by finding images of what you are working toward in life on the Internet.

For example, when asked about your dream car, you might find a photo of a BMW or an Audi. For your dream home, it might be an ocean-front beach house or a country estate. For travel, feature photos of the destinations you'd most love to visit. I think you get the gist!

Some of the questions are more abstract, so use your imagination. That's what this whole activity is about! Find a picture that represents your answer to the question. For example, let's say generosity is a personality trait you'd like to have. A picture of someone doing charitable works or giving away gifts could represent generosity to you. Or, let's say you're struggling to define what 'healthy' means to you; you might select a photo of yourself in peak form for inspiration.

Whatever you do, answer these questions with pictures that really excite and energize you. They should inspire you to vibrate at a higher level and move into flow with life so that you'll more easily summit these mountains and bring your dreams to reality.

Lifestyle Questions:

- What type of car are you driving?
- Where do you live?
- What kind of house?
- What does it look like?
- Do you own a holiday home?
- Do you travel?
- Where do you go?
- What experiences that make you heart race do you want to achieve?
- What other toys do you have…. jet skis, motor bike, boat?
- What do you like to shop for?
- Do you have a nanny, driver or housekeeper?

Relationship Questions:

- How do you want to be described?
- What do you love about yourself?
- What personality traits would you like to have?
- Who are your close friends?
- What do you love about them?
- What do you do together?

- What sort of friend are you?
- What is your relationship like with your family?
- How do you show them that you love them?
- What do you like to spend time doing?
- What does your perfect partner look like?
- What qualities do they have?
- What does your relationship look like?
- How does this make you feel?
- What do you enjoy doing together?
- What sort of a partner are you?

Health Questions:

- What does 'healthy' mean to you?
- Do you exercise?
- What sort of exercise do you enjoy?
- Who do you exercise with?
- What healthy foods do you enjoy?
- How does this healthy lifestyle improve your mind and body?

Save these photos to your Journal in the Quality Mind app, so they're always at your fingertips for a quick boost to remind you of your dreams. You should also save the images into their own folder on your computer.

Activity #4: Meditation — 10-Day Beginners Series

Beta Brainwaves 13-40 Hz
Associated with worry, stress, paranoia, fear, irritability, moodiness, anger. Connected to weakened health and immune system. Fully awake and alert. Nervousness, depression, and anxiety. People spend most of their time in the beta state.

Alpha Brainwaves 7-13 Hz
Meditation and relaxation begins. Effortless creativity flows. Powerful state for memory and super-learning. A harmonious, peaceful state. Habits, fears, and phobias begin to melt away. Tranquility and calm.

Theta Brainwaves 47 Hz
Insight, Intuition, Inspiration. Answers to important questions can be found. Feels like you are floating. A wonderful realm to explore. Dream like imagery. Good for problem solving. Feel more connected to others.

Delta Brainwaves 0-4 Hz
Renewal, healing, rejuvenation. Deep, dreamless sleep. Very Rewarding. Said to be the entrance to non physical states of reality. Best state for immune system function, restoration, and health.

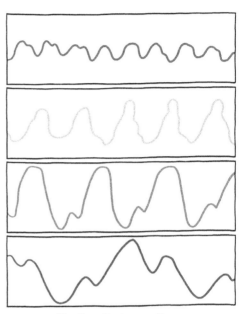

The Four Brainwave States

Brainwaves States

Open your Quality Mind app and navigate to the Meditations tab. You'll discover hundreds of meditations, from those that help you sleep, to those that energize you for a presentation, to walking meditations and more. You'll also find meditations specially calibrated to take you down through each of the brainwave patterns. See graphic above.

What I'd like you to focus on right now, however, is the 10-day Beginners Series of meditations in the app, which I personally walk you through.

This beginner series of meditations will introduce you to and walk you through the basics of regular meditation, and get you accustomed to meditating every day. It's best to make this part of your morning routine, and be sure not to drive or operate machinery during this time.

Once you've completed the 10-day beginners course, you can then progress to the guided meditations.

Case Study: Tiarna Ernst

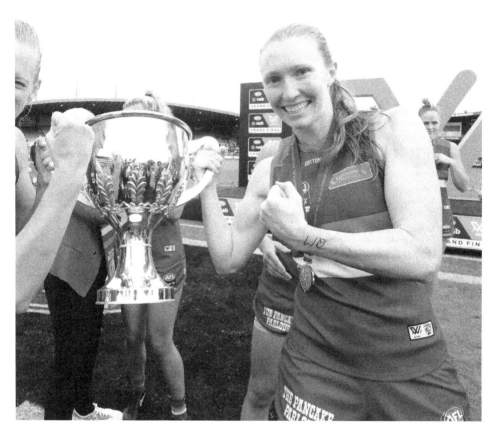

Tiarna Ernst celebrating the Western Bulldogs FC, AFLW, 2018 Championship — Courtesy AFL Photos

Tiarna Ernst is a powerhouse of a human being with two vocations: she is a full-time Obstetrics and Gynecology Advanced Trainee at Royal Brisbane & Women's Hospital, and she also plays for the Gold Coast Suns in the Australian Football League Women's competition.

Tiarna was recruited to the Western Bulldogs in the inaugural draft of the AFLW, where she played all games throughout her three years there and became a Premiership player in 2018. Her debut season with the Suns is set for 2020.

Background: Burning the Candle at Every End

Tiarna is naturally gifted in athleticism and enjoyed dabbling in many different sports as she grew up in a rural community in far north Queensland. While at school, she did track and field followed by some team sports, and she found herself to be successful in her athletic pursuits, even going to national championships in her junior years.

While she always felt like she could achieve something big with sport, she also felt she had to think about her professional career; so she began studying medicine at university. About halfway through her degree, she encountered some women playing AFL across the street from her gym, and she soon started playing footy. She learned the game quickly and soon rose to dominate the local competition.

All of that shifted once she graduated to become a junior doctor. She struggled to balance the demands of working as a new doctor in the health system against her commitments to local footy. AFL wasn't a priority then, but that changed.

"It wasn't until Gillon McLachlan (who is the CEO of the AFL in Australia) announced that there was going to be a women's competition starting in 2017, that I had this idea. I hadn't really pursued my sporting interest to the highest level, but maybe if I tried hard enough and gave it my all, I could actually play AFL Women's next to some of the girls that were considered the best players in Australia at the time."

Tiarna moved to Melbourne to further her career as a doctor, and to train for the AFLW. In her medical career, she struggled to adjust to a new hospital, while also striving to get into a specialist program. She effectively went full-tilt at balancing two high-pressure, full-time jobs: studying and practicing medicine, while simultaneously training for and playing footy. She was determined to be both the best doctor and the best athlete she could be, but it was a struggle.

"I was studying for my specialty exam in a very competitive environment, whilst at the same time playing footy and trying to get drafted," Tiarna explained. "You've got to work for 40-50 hours a week, and you're also trying to train for footy on the weekends and during the week, but then you're also trying to study at least two, three, often four or five hours a day in addition to everything else."

It was an untenable situation, and during that period Tiarna was floundering in a sea of stress and anxiety which impacted her performance at the hospital and on the field. She wasn't coping.

Enter Quality Mind

When Tiarna first met with Richard, she cried the entire time. "I think it was just this huge amount of pressure and stress, and I just let it all out. That's all I can remember — it was just all spilling out. Obviously, he could see the impact the stress and pressures were having on my life." Richard immediately said, "Look, I can help you," and he went on to explain that she had to commit 100% to the program for it to work. 50% wouldn't do it. Tiarna was at a tipping point, with vicious crocs on one side and a Quality Mind on the other. She was in.

The biggest impact that the Quality Mind program had on Tiarna is that it eliminated all sense of those pressures she was drowning in before. Acknowledging that there's a stress problem in the medical industry — that medical students learn from overworked and stressed-out doctors until they internalize and perpetuate the same needless anxiety — Tiarna realized that she was worrying about things she couldn't control.

"Once I started to recognize the differences in channeling your energy and channeling your thoughts — by not having to worry about any of the pressures, it made work one, so much easier; two, a lot more enjoyable; and three, it almost became addictive. I was no longer going to let all the stress and chaos, and even the medical emergencies that happen at work, affect me. It became addictive to not let any of those external influences impact how I was feeling, how I was acting and how I was channeling my energies."

By mastering her mind and living in the now, the art of balancing work and footy was no longer a burden. "I just let it happen. I just floated through work. Things came my way, I dealt with them, and I didn't have to worry or stress about what had happened in the past or what was going to happen in the future." She also credits Quality Mind with making her a better doctor, giving her the tools to cope with the demands of her profession and avoiding burn out.

After joining the Quality Mind program, Tiarna's game also improved so much that she was drafted into the AFLW, and her record of frequent injury ended.

Busting a Kidney

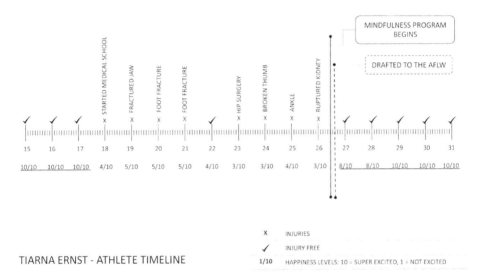

TIARNA ERNST - ATHLETE TIMELINE

Tiarna Ernst Self Assessed Timeline

Looking over Tiarna's timeline, we can see where she started out playing with love for the game — her reported happiness was 10/10 in junior play. Once she started medical school, however, and life became more serious, her energy tanked and injuries started piling up, right up through to an exhibition match she played as part of the Melbourne Demons in 2015.

"I was obviously trying to get drafted in 2017, and I had an opportunity to play at Etihad Stadium (now Marvel Stadium) in one of the first exhibition series in the lead-up to the inaugural AFL Women's competition, and in that game I actually ruptured my kidney.

"At the time we were down, we were losing, and just before the start of the second quarter, we'd just got a bit of a spray from our coach at quarter time," Tiarna explained. "I felt like I hadn't done very much in the game, and I think I started to worry over all the things that had happened, so I was focused on the past. I was down on myself because

I hadn't really played very well in that last quarter, and I knew I needed to play better than this other ruck, who at the time was beating me."

"Those thoughts meant that, when I went up into the contest, I went about the motion of being in the ruck in a different manner than I usually do. I didn't protect myself, or protect my abdomen, and that's how I got a knee to the belly: I started thinking about my opponent and things that had happened before, rather than focusing on right there and then, and what I needed to do. I was all out of flow."

Tiarna was no stranger to injury, having faced a fractured jaw, fractured feet, a broken thumb, and more, but the ruptured kidney stands out. She played the rest of the game, only to be taken to hospital later where a CT scan revealed the extent of her injury. "It was a devastating injury that took six months for me to recover from," she said. "Since that injury though, I haven't had any more. I started the Quality Mind journey with Richard, and since then I've played every AFL Women's game from the start of the competition and I haven't missed any trainings. It's all because of my ability to use the program to channel my energy where I've needed it to make sure that I remain injury-free and not impacted by pressures and stress around me."

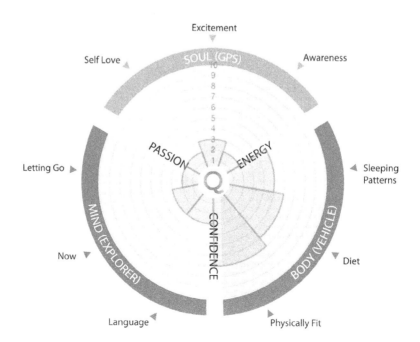

Figure 1: Tiarna Ernst Before her QM journey began – Injured & Inconsistent Performances

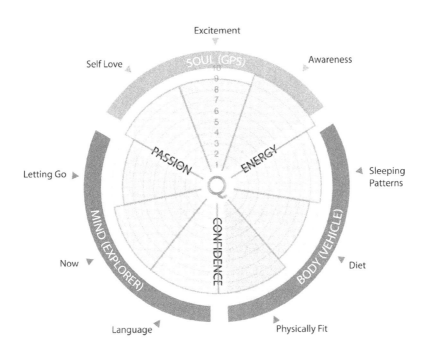

Figure 2: Tiarna Ernst During her QM journey — Injury-Free & Consistent Performances

Creating the Time

When Tiarna began the program, she found it difficult to figure out where she was going to find the time in her days to do the program. While challenging at first, the program is so organic that it became a natural part of her day, especially with the development of the app. "The app has made it more efficient and convenient, so that you can do it throughout the day; and you have those little reminders and coaching steps."

Creating the space for meditation was vital for Tiarna's transformation, given the high pressures surrounding her at work and play. "Just having that moment to stop and have absolute silence was very therapeutic for me. I needed that break, while filling every other minute of my day constantly balancing work, then footy." Owning that peace helped Tiarna become invigorated and allowed her to deliberately direct her energy where it was needed — toward her highest excitement.

The skills she developed with Quality Mind also allowed her to confront and dissolve limiting beliefs around her sports performance, particularly those beliefs insisting she couldn't balance a professional career with a sports career. And while tackling these limiting beliefs has taken time, and may require later redress, working through them has had a remarkable impact on her performance.

The Final Goal

When asked where she would be without Quality Mind, Tiarna is unequivocal.

"I would've burnt out. Quality Mind was really the main thing that helped me get to that level where I continued working as a full-time doctor as well as actually being drafted. Without it, I don't think I would have been drafted. Since I started the program in 2015, it has contributed to every success I've had so far, both sporting and professional — and with that has also come new career opportunities."

Would Tiarna recommend the Quality Mind program to everyone?

"Yes, absolutely. I think it works in all areas of life, in all career areas. The main thing is that you have to be committed to it; you can't just try and do it once or twice a week. It ends up being a daily thing that becomes a routine, that then transforms the way that you use your energy throughout your life — and that can mean success wherever you feel you want to achieve success."

To access Tiarna's full video testimonial please go to the Quality Mind Website: www.qualitymindglobal.com/success-stories/videos

Step #3: Clean

Even in our earliest days, we're infected with limiting beliefs — those ideas that make our world smaller and meaner, with limited possibilities.

We move through this human experience accepting, believing and buying into limiting beliefs from our parents, our leaders, our societies, our cultures and our media. We're being covered with a layer of restrictive muck every day, but because it's not visible to the naked eye, most of us never wash it off.

Throughout our childhood and adolescence, we're like sponges: absorbing and recording everything we hear and see, but not consciously analyzing it. We don't have those skills yet, which is too bad because this is also when we are developing and designing our unique identity. Since our lives as children are controlled by our family and those who care for us, we usually have their belief systems, actions, and behaviors pushed upon us. We're literally being programmed and shaped with their software.

We are all born with naked purity and naturally high vibrations; however, as the years progress, we inevitably find ourselves rolling around in mud with our energies diluted. We're also told that we'll become our parents, or that the apple doesn't fall far from the tree, or that it is our duty to emulate the thoughts and actions of another authority figure. If you're happy with that, you can continue it, but you certainly don't have to. In order for us not to carry on and perpetuate the same attitudes and beliefs of our predecessors, we must identify what beliefs do not service us and then eliminate those beliefs from our lives. That's the sole focus of this next step of our Quality Mind process: CLEAN.

Remember, up until around age 16, our whole existence is focused around making sure we are safe. The Child's mind rules the roost, ensuring that we have all of our necessary safety mechanisms firmly in place. We know when to cross the street, when not to touch things that are too hot, how to avoid dangerous situations, and more. Once we've reached the middle of our teenage years, we've accepted that we're safe in everyday life and we're ready to move on. However, by this stage you are living with a powerful Child's mind that doesn't recognise any need for change, whilst also living with a collection of ingrained bad habits and limiting beliefs. So essentially, your path up the mountain has been ambushed before you've even started, despite your best intentions.

Let's say you visit a coal mine, and before you descend into the mine, the occupational health and safety manager says, "You need to put on a safety suit along with these goggles, mask and shoes." The suit and every piece of gear he hands you is bright white and pristine. The manager continues, "We're going to walk down this tunnel, and we're not going to touch the sides. In fact, we're not going to do anything. We're just going to walk down the tunnel, and at the end we'll walk out of the tunnel."

You put this beautifully clean white suit on, and you walk through the tunnel as requested. When you emerge, however, you discover your suit is not so clean anymore. You're dirty and you're covered in black soot. And yet, you never even touched the sides — you simply walked down the middle of the mine shaft.

So that's life in a nutshell. It's a big, dirty mine shaft! We walk through life and we take on all of these limiting belief systems without doing anything. Perhaps family tells us that we're less than we are, so we tear ourselves down in our own minds. We may misread another person and when they don't react as we predict, we get insulted by their behavior. There could be game replays or player interviews on television that we get dramatically involved with which impacts our energy. The coach might have given us a hard time. These sorts of things all stick to us and they've got to be cleaned off.

So, at the end of the day, take off your white protective suit, then wash it down and prepare it for the next day. If you don't, you'll find yourself dragging a dirty suit through life: the filters get clogged up, the dirt gets through the goggles, and suddenly all that muck is in your eyes and it's in your mind. It's impacting how you perceive reality, which means it's changing your reality into something miserable and squalid.

It's a standard part of everyone's daily life to shower — or, at least, wash our face and brush our teeth and put on clean clothes. Cleaning our physical bodies is common and expected, as it should be. But do we clean our minds down at least once a day? Not many people do. Even if they are doing some daily cleaning, they're most often doing meditation alone. Meditation is fantastic, and it's a key part of our program, but it's only about 10% of the daily cleaning process. Meditation is just one tool in our Quality Mind toolbox, and there's more to do if you want to keep yourself clean enough to shine like a beacon of light.

The goal is to clean away everything you've taken on from others, and to be left with the raw and unadulterated energy sources that we all share at birth: love, self-acceptance, empathy and self-expression.

We each carry a light inside of ourselves. For many, that inner candle is dimming. For some, their candles have just about been snuffed out. It's up to us to keep our candle burning brightly, both feeding on and providing high energy, enthusiasm, and excitement. Cleaning down is the key — making sure our candles are kept in polished lanterns with pristine glass that amplify our light.

When you clean yourself down, the raw energy inside of you emanates like a beacon, and you'll quickly discover that you're highly attractive to others. People respond to your light because it reminds them of their own, and allows them to discover that their own light is still burning within them. People love that feeling, that wave of inspiration that whispers in their own voices, "I could be like that." This enthusiasm is infectious. The more you clean down, the more brightly you shine, the more you ignite others, and that's when we can change the world — when we emit that intoxicating energy that make others feel like sunshine.

Cleaning out your filters daily changes the neurons in your brain, which changes the superhighways in your mind, and ultimately results in a change in your identity. This new 2.0 version of you that you're creating has a much brighter, focused view of the future. This upward shift in energy is clear as day to others, as well. When you're in a meeting or speaking to someone, you'll discover you have an edge in getting others to listen to you. You're more likely to make a deal, get a job, or secure a sports role — all because you're burning so brightly and other people respond to that very favorably.

Elite athletes will quickly understand that cleaning down is one of the most important parts of the Quality Mind process, and that it's not just a job that gets finished. Cleaning is a process that you must maintain forever, because we're all living in a world designed to pollute our world view and choke out our lights. We're still walking through that coal mine in our pristine white suits — so keep your lantern shining brightly, and you'll find yourself lighting hundreds of other candles along the way.

At this point in the Quality Mind process, your influence and leadership qualities go through the roof, and you inspire others to fan their own lights. This is the pinnacle of power for the elite athlete today: they can become national and global influencers, giving the most incredible gift anyone could receive by helping others shine their lights more brightly across the world.

Limiting Beliefs

We've covered Thought Shopping, which is used for quick mental transformation. You identify how you're feeling, and if your vibrational levels are in a negative space, you select a new thought to refocus you into a state of higher energy. This in turn reinforces the remapping of your neurons.

When you're dealing with belief systems, however, you'll need to bring out the big guns. Limiting beliefs can be heavier and stickier than single thoughts. They don't want to simply disappear, and they often require a more dedicated focus.

Remember: a belief is simply a thought that you keep thinking, which makes it a belief.

These belief systems tend to hide in the dark corners of your mind, taking refuge in the shadows. They don't want to be recognized, defined, and purged. These beliefs are the domain of the Child's mind, and as you now know, the Child doesn't want to lose control of the center stage! When you're drilling down to focus on your beliefs, be aware that they'll hide from you. They don't come up that quickly much of the time. If you're fully aware and focused on how you're thinking and feeling each day, however, you'll find limiting beliefs pop up organically like a splinter. A deep splinter can remain in your body for years, and may require serious work to remove. Limiting beliefs are no different.

Just take a look at a few common limiting beliefs and how they're first embedded. In my case, my mother told me when I was young, "You're not very good at maths. You're just like me." That became one of my belief systems, and this isn't a unique example. How many of us have heard something similar and internalized it? Then we suffer in school or somewhere else in life, and who can say what opportunities we've missed out on because someone programmed us with this belief that then became part of our identity without us realizing it.

Another limiting belief we commonly pick up from our families is classism — "the rich are arrogant and greedy" or "the poor are lazy and deserve what they get" — and racism and sexism. These beliefs structures are deeply and directly harmful to our lives and to our world. You probably won't get rich, for example, if you have an underlying bias that rich people are assholes! Just look at people who win the lottery, or at so many pro athletes that make it big. They make millions of dollars, but so often they just can't hold on to it, and they may even end up bankrupt. This is why it's so important to clean down our minds and clean out these harmful or unproductive belief systems on a regular basis. We must design our future selves with deliberation, focus, and excitement.

The fact of life is that we're all going to die, but you've got this one opportunity to live your best potential as we take this masterclass of masterclasses together. We're giving you the tools to jettison all the grief, misery, and trash thinking that is weighing you down, and we're showing you exactly how to uncover the raw power you already possess. And the answers to all of your questions are already within you! You don't need to purchase a new self; you've just got to clean what's already there.

Once you awaken that bright light that's currently dimmed within you, you'll uncover pure intelligence and raw energy that will get you back in flow with life, enabling you to shine brighter and achieve your biggest dreams. That's what you came here to do, to go within and find that potential that you've been missing. If you don't go within, you'll go without.

The Four Stages of Diffusing Old Beliefs

Let me first reiterate that a belief is simply a thought that gets repeated over and over until it wears a groove in your mind and becomes accepted as a BELIEF or a fact. It then becomes a part of your identity, and sometimes it's even a formative piece of your identity if it's implanted early enough. The great news is that you don't need to keep any beliefs that are not helping you. There is a four stage process that will enable you to get rid of them.

Desire

The first stage in changing a belief is having the *desire* to do so. It's as simple as that. You must have the deepest interest in making this change, and be fundamentally committed to wanting it. This burning desire often emerges once someone gets fed up with life, and just throws up their hands, either literally or metaphorically, while exclaiming, "Right. I'm done with this."

Remember, when you're not listening to your Master mind, you're going to get contrast in your life, and if you're in a position where life isn't working for you, that contrast will come through. If you're not in alignment with who you really are and what you're here to do, that contrast will come through again, and it often manifests as unhappiness, injury, or disease.

At this point, you'll realize, "Okay, I need to change my belief systems" because you're creating your current reality. Once you've identified that desire to change, hold on to that inner passion.

Definition

The second stage is *defining the belief* that you want to change, and understanding why it needs to go. It's likely to be a belief you've purchased for free, or borrowed from family, friends, the media or society surrounding you. This belief has served you up until now as well — otherwise, you wouldn't have it. Recognize the ways in which it's been of benefit to you, and define why you no longer require that benefit.

Dedication

In the third stage, you are building the *dedication* to purge the belief. There may be a good amount of internal discussion, or even discussion with a mentor or confidante, as you clearly define who you want to be and how the current belief does not fit into that new version of you.

Examine your behaviors, reflect on your beliefs, and see how the belief you'd like to excise interacts with the rest of your internal ecosystem. Firm up your dedication to defining and becoming who you want to be, until you can say, without hesitation, "I'm ready to be the next version of me."

Detachment

The fourth and final stage is *detachment* of the belief. Once you have expressed a desire to change, defined what needs to change, and show dedication to becoming the new you, it's time to compassionately release the belief that no longer benefits you.

Don't beat yourself up over having the belief in the first place. Don't think of the belief you're letting go of as wholly representative of you as a person. Simply understand that the belief was part of the old you, and because you're always changing, you can let that piece go without shame or regret. Every moment of every day, right down to the cellular level, you are always changing. Detach yourself from the past and move into the new you.

Activity #5: Remove Limiting Beliefs Meditation

To assist you through this process, open the Quality Mind app on your mobile device and navigate to the Meditations tab. Look for the 'Remove Limiting Beliefs' meditation.

This is a 15-minute meditation that I recorded, which will walk you through a relaxation and visualization exercise to help you release these beliefs no longer benefiting you.

This is a meditation that you'll wish to return to regularly as you purge those old beliefs to make room for the new you. Once you locate an old belief, follow the 8 Step Belief Busting Questionnaire to eliminate it instantly.

1. Is this belief statement 100% true? yes or no
2. What does holding onto this belief give you?
3. What has this belief already cost you so far?
4. What is it costing you right now?
5. If you hold on to it, what will this belief cost you in 1-5 years?
6. Who would you become and how would you act without this old belief?
7. What's the exact opposite of this belief?
8. Once you have the statement that is the exact opposite of this belief then — SAY IT, FEEL IT and BE IT! Until you own it!

What You Think is What You Get

The single most effective way to ensure frustration in your future is to be constantly frustrated and worried about elements of your current life. It's as simple as that: your thoughts become your reality. Harboring negative belief systems and allowing negative thought patterns to persist allows an unfulfilled and stagnant life to become a self-fulfilling prophecy.

When you have negative expectations, you're creating a space where the only possible outcome — or even understanding — is negative. When you define something as wrong, that thing can only be experienced as wrong. That will never change so long as you continue within the same mindset without cleaning out your filters and deliberately changing your mindset.

You're the one creating your own frustration. You're creating your own definition of what's dissatisfying about your life, and you're the one defining what's out of alignment with your highest excitement. For an elite athlete, there is nothing as devastating in the game or out of it as frustration — especially when you know that you haven't been playing at your highest level.

To stop this frustration from mounting, you've got to create something else: a way of looking at the world that doesn't create needless negativity. The idea is to understand that wherever you are in any given moment — even if it's not where you prefer to be, it's where you need to be to learn what you need to learn, even if you don't prefer it.

Everything is neutral until you give it meaning. Realize the difference between neutrally recognizing that you don't prefer something, and tainting your life with negativity by negatively defining the experience. Once you validate an experience, it'll stick to you like glue because you're giving it undue attention and power. What keeps you in this self-perpetuating cycle of frustration is defining what's going on around you as an invalid experience that shouldn't be happening. You created that experience. You defined it. You gave it a negative vibration and discarded what you could have learned. Ultimately, you are invalidating yourself — and you'll find yourself manifesting the same challenges and frustrations again and again as you feel invalidated and constricted.

Everything is just a mirror. Are you seeing frowning faces and concern being reflected back at you? Then you know you're not validating yourself because that frown is coming from your own face. Hence why, in the next reflection model, we encourage you to put your face on the faces of those surrounding you, so that you can appreciate the real lesson in what you're experiencing, instead of seeing the other person as the problem. You'll receive the real lesson, and you can recognize through the frown that you don't prefer what is happening. Don't validate it, just thank the frown and turn it upside down.

Now you're smiling because that's what you prefer. You've taken the gift of those frowns and discovered the element inside of you that wasn't in alignment with where you wanted to be. Decide to smile at everything that happens. You know it's going to serve you in a positive way, because it's up to you!

As you step into becoming the creator, it's critical that you understand that any frustration with or invalidation of a belief system is within you. Everything around you is reflecting what you project out into the world. As you design the new you, treat every situation in a positive way, and find the good in every opportunity. Things are going to happen in your existence that you don't prefer: you may get sacked from a job you love, or break up with a significant other you weren't planning to leave, or struggle with your financial situation not matching what you'd like, but none of those experiences is innately negative. There's probably a better job for you, or your life partner waiting right around the corner, or a financial windfall just a short time away if you maintain a positive outlook in life.

This happens with small things as well, like going through your daily travels. Let's say your flight gets bumped, but then you get upgraded on the next flight. Or discovering you left your wallet at home when you're out for lunch, only to discover a forgotten twenty in your jacket pocket. When you're cooling your heels at the airport or wondering whether someone will pay for your lunch, you'll be tempted to throw your hands in the air and say, "it figures." Ignore that; it doesn't. Instead, put your hands in the air and say, "It's happening for the right reasons." Then allow the gift to come through.

Can you maintain your energy and your focus? If you're not committed to doing so, there's no point in doing this program. If your mind is constantly worried about the next thing that's going to go wrong, things are just going to constantly go wrong for you. Where your focus goes, your energy flows. It's the choice of each athlete and each person to recognize and understand the power they have within themselves. As soon as you develop a belief system around certain aspects or elements in life, that belief system is going to play out in front of you again and again, whether you like it or not — good, bad, or neutral.

Your Mirror Reflection

Imagine that you were dropped down on planet Earth by yourself, and you were expected to go through this human experience alone. If that was the case, it would be extremely difficult (if not impossible) for you to actually learn anything of significance, other than how the trees grow and the tides flow. You would be hard pressed to learn that the whole human experience is about growth and self-expression and evolving the soul.

Thankfully, we're not alone here on planet Earth, and we share our journey to experience, create, manifest, and understand ourselves better with over seven billion other people. And on the journey to understanding ourselves better, the quickest and most powerful way to learn more is through others.

In this conceptual framework, everyone is the center of their own you-universe. As the planetary center, a number of satellites revolve in orbit around you. Think about satellites in our world: there are thousands of satellites orbiting the planet Earth, deliberately put there to be a reflection tool (in a very simplistic sense). For example, if a television station in Japan wants to beam a program throughout the world, it bounces the transmission off a satellite (or multiple satellites) until the transmission is reflected back to Earth. The satellites are acting as mirrors, reflecting what is sent out to them.

So if we are the center of our own metaphorical universe, our metaphorical satellites are other people — people like our family members, partners, friends, work colleagues, and so on. The things that these satellites are reflecting back to us represent the lessons necessary for our own self-growth. They're offering us gold; they're offering us the keys to become our true selves.

What are your satellites reflecting back to you? Is the group of people around you triggering frustration or inspiration, or perhaps both? Meditate or tap into your intuition on why you're responding with those feelings in order to grasp the lesson standing in front of you. Perhaps there's an area within you that needs to be fulfilled or discarded.

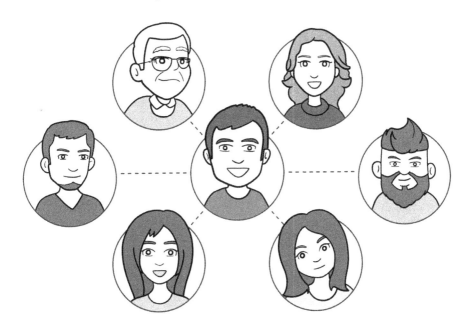

Your Mirror Reflections

Let's say that you're frustrated with your mother, and what you're frustrated about is that she doesn't understand you. You're constantly arguing with her, or there's a persistent feeling of uneasiness between you. If that's the case, then there's an area within you that is unsettled and needs to be examined. You need to shine that light within yourself to identify that area for growth, because it's that need for personal development driving the contrast that's manifesting within your relationship with your mother.

Do you have a real problem with a teammate? Maybe you feel they're too arrogant, or that they aren't taking their role as seriously as they should. Consider what it is about your own sports performance that is making you feel uncertain, and redirect your energies toward firming up your training and improving team cohesion.

Of course, it can be difficult to separate our personal feelings for other people from the lessons that they may represent for us — especially if you're getting contrast in the form of frustration with people around you. Luckily, we have a simple exercise to help you quickly cut through your personal feelings and focus only on the mirror image.

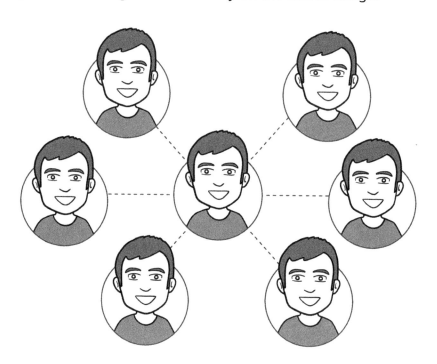

Mirror Reflection Activity

To get started, close your eyes. Visualize that person and the frustration you have with them, then put your own face on their face in your mind's eye. Once you identify them with yourself, ask yourself: what is the challenge here? What lesson am I missing, or what do I need to get from this relationship?

Proceed to have a mental conversation with yourself, pretending that the other person is actually you. Every issue that you have is actually you, so the issues you think you're having with someone else, you're actually having with yourself.

All of the people surrounding you are quite simply reflecting the gifts and opportunities that are within you; they're deliberately designed for your own growth in every capacity. There's no such thing as coincidence with those people who revolve through your life.

I refer us again to my early life: as a young man in my late teens, I was quite angry because of my misinterpretation of existence. Frustrations with my outer world impacted my inner world; the more heated and frustrated my inner world became, the more I attracted that same level of aggression in the outer world. I got into quite a few bar fights and outright brawls, and a bit of trouble with the law. I was consistently creating my own reality of strife because I was not listening to my outer world or seeing the lessons I needed to learn reflected in those around me. I was completely in the grasp of my Child's mind.

Once we bring ourselves into alignment with our surroundings and truly open our eyes, we elevate ourselves to a new level of awareness. We can see the opportunities and gifts being offered to us through our experiences and our relationships.

Look at school: you go through grade one, two, three, and so forth, but you cannot advance to the next level until you've demonstrated your knowledge of the current level. Many people are consistently having the same types of arguments with their family members for multiple years because they are not advancing. They are still playing the same record over and over in their head, and until they change the music, they'll be stuck in grade one, singing the same old song! They're unable to see the gift being offered by this contrast, and so they're unable to grasp it, and they repeat the same mistakes.

Inner World VS Outer World

Once someone has progressed far enough to look within themselves, there's a process of building their systems back up on a solid foundation of self-worth. As they open up the connection with their intuitive minds and access the system of the whole human experience, you'll see the pressure valves of the mind open wider and wider. They're taking in lessons and expelling steam; they're centering themselves, and breathing deeply without feeling heavy pressure from the outer world.

You can easily see why building towards that level of power within the system is so important for athletes in particular, as they're consistently under high levels of pressure. When they're not standing on a solid foundation and the winds of change come sweeping through (as they always do), that's when you get knocked over, whether by illness or injury.

The mind must be built on a firm foundation from the inside out. Assess the outer world, use it to shine a light on your interior, and then ensure that your inner world is growing through understanding as you nurture self-worth and forgiveness. Acknowledge the outer world for what it is, then let it go. You know full well that 95% of society are living in their Child's mind most of the time, which gives you a level of logical leverage to take the world as it is: you can't negotiate with a 12 or 13 year old.

You can, however, understand the actions of those still living mainly within their Child's mind. This makes it easier to focus on forgiveness, empathy and compassion within all the relationships that surround you. Don't hold on to any negativity, whether in work, business, life, or at home. Keep the lesson, and release the past. Recognize every current relationship, every ending relationship, and every former relationship for the perfect gifts they are or were, complete in their times.

Remember, if you're struggling to take this practice to the highest level, just see everyone as you. They're all you in disguise, and we're all helping each other find opportunities for growth. As they say, we are all ONE at the end of the day.

You can't remain at the level where you're pointing your finger constantly at other people, saying they're the problem, they're the issue, and not taking any responsibility for your own actions and thoughts.

That is a level of negative growth. The people you point out will continue to frustrate you, or they'll leave and you'll find yourself surrounded by new relationships that frustrate you the same way. You can't change the reflection until you change the source within you.

After my parents' separation and my failed attempt at playing elite football for the AFL, I was experiencing major frustrations — and that's putting it mildly! So I decided to escape interstate and play for teams around the country. I thought running away would be the answer to all my problems and that a new environment would make things better, but I just started seeing the same problems facing me no matter where I turned — until I turned toward my inner world.

I started to appreciate that my outer world was a reflection of my inner world, and then I discovered myself surrounded by all these gifts. The point is that your problems will always follow you, because your issues are you, and you can't run away from yourself! That's the secret to really understanding your outer world. Sit down, face yourself and the world around you, and be completely aware of what's triggering you at every opportunity, throughout every day.

Why is Understanding Our DNA Important?

Deoxyribonucleic acid (DNA) is a nucleic acid that contains the genetic instructions for the development and function of living things. All known cellular life and some viruses contain DNA. The main role of DNA in the cell is the long-term storage of information. DNA quite simply is the crowning glory of existence.

The basis of who we are comes from lineage of our DNA, and that we cannot change. It's simply our framework, and our ancestors never had access to the evolutionary tools (such as mind training) that we have access to today. So it's now our time and our responsibility to change the code. This is necessary because the old code has viruses and needs an upgrade, because we are aware that there is a code, and because we now have access to the tools for change. The world, and individuals, have not (for the most part) been heading in the right direction. You just need to watch the news!

We don't want future generations to carry the same lineage of destruction, greed and harmfulness that currently exists around the world, and while we can't change the past, we can change the future. So the first thing we can do to create massive change is to clean ourselves down. From there we can then assist in cleaning others, and in cleaning the world, thus changing our code and the codes of others. Awareness of our DNA is first, and once we understand who we are and where we have come from, we can assess our family belief systems and whether or not they are actually working for us.

Activity #6: How Do I Recode Myself?

You recode yourself by wanting to understand yourself and why you are who you are. This is a fantastic and enlightening activity. You need to pick 3 members of your family, preferably up line: mother, father, grandparents, and if not possible, you can fall back on aunties and uncles. We want to find out what pain, joy, limiting beliefs and empowering assumptions of those that came before you carried and transmitted to you and your DNA.

It's best to ask all the questions, however you choose. Please upload your answers here on your Journal.

1. What is your favourite childhood memory?
2. If you could ask 1 question to both your mum and dad, what would it be?
3. Is there any history of anxiety, depression or trauma in the family lineage?
4. What has been your history or beliefs about accumulating money?
5. Are there any family secrets you haven't told me about?
6. What do you think is the biggest gift you got from your parents and how are you implementing it in your life?
7. How would you rate your relationship with your parents?
8. What have been your 3 biggest challenges in life so far?
9. If you could start your life again, what would you do differently?
10. What was your highest excitement/dream that you didn't get to realise?

Understanding your history is one way to greatly accelerate the personal path of enlightenment and expanded consciousness. By shining a light on why we may be the way we are, we can empower ourselves, increase our awareness and alter our behavior to create alternate outcomes. The more you clean down and shed light on who you are, the more you activate new levels of energy and clarity in everyday living.

Love & Forgiveness

Forgiveness of yourself and forgiveness of others is critical and essential if you are to progress and move forward.

We all make mistakes and we must make amends and fix our relationships, both with ourselves and with others. Remember, every issue (is-you) and it's an opportunity for growth, so see it that way! We will always encounter some level of conflict, disappointment or disharmony in our lives from time to time. It's how we handle this, and how we take ownership and move on from it that dictates how we feel in the moments and days that follow. Forgiveness will quite literally set you free!

For those that continually jump the hurdles of forgiveness, they will find that their relationships are stronger and more meaningful than ever before, both with themselves and with others.

Activity #7: Questions to Reveal the Gifts of Your Reflection to Love & Forgive

Make a list of all the people you need to love and forgive to take another big step forward into your future self, and apply these questions to each of them, one at a time:

1. Who is the person you have the issue (is-you) with?
2. Within 10 words, what is the problem you are experiencing with them?
3. Within 10 words, why is it bothering you right now?
4. What is the reflection gifting you right now, so you can learn from it and advance yourself?

If you have the answers, close your eyes, hug them and thank them for the gift.

5. If you did not get the answer, then close your eyes, take 3 deep breaths, sit back and relax. Now replace the person's face with your own face, so you are looking at yourself, and ask yourself what areas do you need to work on for YOU to become whole?

Ask and allow, and it will come through, either now or in the near future if you are genuinely prepared for the answer.

6. So now, what are the holes which you need to fill within yourself to become whole?
7. In case you didn't find the gift again ask yourself — "how would I react as my Master if that person was a 5 year old child?" Then go back to question 2 and start the process again.

Case Study: Easton Wood

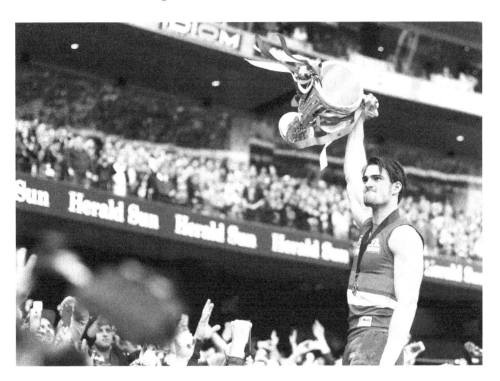

Easton Wood celebrates the 2017 WBFC, AFL Premiership / Championship. — Courtesy AFL Photos

Introduction

Easton Wood has been an elite athlete in the Australian Football League (AFL) for 12 years, and he is still going strong. He grew up in country Australia, where he began dreaming of playing sport professionally from a very young age. Just two weeks after finishing high school, his boyhood dream was realised when he was drafted to the Western Bulldogs FC (WBFC). He was just 18 at the time.

When he arrived at the Bulldogs in 2007, Easton instantly became prone to many injuries, which he found both frustrating and perplexing, since this had never been the case in his many years of playing footy growing up.

"In our football league we play 22 games a year, and I probably would have missed about 80 games in the first 5 years through repeat hamstring injuries. I felt like my career was slipping away because of all the injuries and related issues."

The Turning Point

"In 2013, I again had a big hamstring injury and I missed almost an entire season. That was my turning point, and this also coincided with when I started working with Richard. It was during rehabbing that hamstring. I had another year to go on my contract, and I thought, if I don't show anything in this last year, I probably won't get another contract. So I jumped right in with both feet."

"I'd worked with Richard for a number of years previously when he was the Leadership & Culture Coach at WBFC where he was running and facilitating leadership and culture programs for our entire football club. So Richard was well aware of me and my struggles as an athlete and he recognized my potential as well. He felt that I wasn't quite reaching that potential because of my mind. So I backed him, and I backed myself, and I started the QM program."

First Encounters

"First encounters of Richard, he's unbelievably driven and he's incredibly, incredibly passionate. I've met a lot of people in the sports industry, and he's probably one of the most driven and passionate of all of them. He made it clear that he believed I had untapped potential, and if I didn't act now I could lose my chance to recognise it. I whole-heartedly agreed with him, and he was great in helping me reach that realization."

"When I was first introduced to the Quality Mind program, I thought it was refreshingly different. We weren't doing anything like that in the team space, we weren't focusing on the way we prepare our mind. It just wasn't a done thing in our team, or something we've ever worked on week to week. It was obviously quite different in that regard."

"Once I began the program, it helped me gain control over the inevitable stress of the game. Something I hadn't dealt with really well at all in the early years of my career! The one thing you can guarantee in professional sport is that stress and pressure is going to be a constant, and you need to learn effective ways to deal with that. The Quality Mind program helped me to understand that, and to develop the tools to deal with that ongoing stress and pressure."

"The program also really helped me to understand myself better, and it encouraged me to explore certain things about myself that I wouldn't have explored prior."

"I believe that in understanding myself and in becoming aware of where the pressure, the stress and the anxiety of playing football was really coming from, I was able to make lasting changes in my mindset. I finally understood that my frequent injuries were like self-fulfilling prophecies. I was expecting to be injured, and it had become an ugly cycle."

"Once I managed to get my head around what was really going on, I was then able to control it a whole lot better, and alleviate that stress, and alleviate that pressure. It was getting out of the way of the fears, and the stress, and the pressure that was holding me back, and understanding it, learning how to deal with it, and then controlling it so I could finally reach my full potential as an athlete. As a result, I didn't have that stress in my system and I've been injured a lot less since. Even after completing the program and completing my time with Richard, I have the tools and the knowledge, so the results are continuing."

"One of the most challenging things was understanding and accepting that I was my own worst enemy. I was putting the stress and the pressure on myself, and that was having a negative effect physically. At first it was confronting and challenging for me to get my head around that. As soon as I did, though, I started to see some really positive outcomes. People just have to be willing to be uncomfortable and willing to have a go and explore new ideas."

From 2013 to the end of 2015, Easton worked directly and privately with Richard & the QM program. In this time Easton won the Club Best and Fairest, and he was selected All-Australian in 2015. In 2016 Easton captained the team to a winning premiership.

To access Easton's full video testimonial please go to the Quality Mind Website: www.qualitymindglobal.com/success-stories/videos

Step #4: Dream

Discovering Synchronicity

When you are connecting to what's really exciting you in life, you are also connecting to your Master mind. Your intuition, your GPS, your soul — communicates to you in many ways, but most evidently through your excitement. If you're aligned with your purpose, your passion, and you're excited by your everyday existence and where you're heading in life, then you're in flow with life.

Your Master mind also talks to you through imagination. For instance, think of a moment when you've woken up or been in the shower and experienced a sudden vision of what you want to do with your life. This vision represents a powerful idea for your life that fills your heart with excitement and energy. You really feel that that's where you want to go. You really feel that's what you want to create for your life. It's this full-throttle excitement that confirms your vision is possible. What so often happens next though, is that your vision moves from the heart space, where passion comes from, up to the mind, which is full of limiting beliefs, fear, and worry. Your feeling of excitement can then become diluted and gets largely filtered out. You forget about that shining vision of opportunity, even though your hearts intuition — which has its own powerful mind — has already told you, "You can do that."

Your Master mind is always communicating with you through your excitement levels, through your imagination, and through synchronicity. Synchronicity is that concept defined by Carl Jung, in which meaningful connections exist between two events that don't seem to have an apparent connection. A synchronicity might appear or feel like a mere happen chance which is in perfect alignment with your current thoughts or ideas. For example, you may be thinking about someone you haven't seen or thought about for years, only to bump into them that very same day, or you decide you want to start a business and you randomly meet someone that specialises in that field that same week.

Synchronicity is another way that your Master mind signals you're moving in the right direction. It's a magnificent indication that you are on the right track! If you're in flow with life and you're excited by where you're going, if you know that you're living out your purpose and your passion, then you'll be more aware of the synchronicity of an encounter and that will accelerate you toward what you want at a faster rate.

Synchronicity will always be at play as it is another universal law; however, if you're vibrating high and you have a positive outlook, you will be more inclined to read the play!

Recognizing Contrast

In regards to the Master mind, there is no right or wrong. Sure, we live in a dualistic world: Up, down. Yes, no. Left, right. Yet when it comes to right or wrong, there really is no right or wrong — there's just what you've created. Everything is perfect and in flow with what you've created and what you are creating.

Contrast is quite simply the guiding hand of the higher mind providing you with more choices and moving you in different directions. Your Master mind is always guiding you on the path of least resistance, and because we've been equipped with the keys of self-creation and we are ultimately in charge of our choices, we can often find ourselves going off course. And because our Master mind sees our life from the top of the mountain well before we do, it will know when something needs to change, which can cause anxiety. Most people don't like change!

Contrast will help guide you — and sometimes (most of the time) we don't want it to, because change can be scary. Contrast will often occur when things aren't working in your favour. Contrast might occur when a relationship isn't working out, when a job is about to finish (that you didn't want to finish), when finances are a struggle, or when you're getting some other element of pressure in your inner or outer world. Contrast is a gift — disguised as pain or discomfort, or illness — that is guiding you in a different direction from the one in which you're travelling. But because we are mostly control freaks, we find contrast difficult to allow in, so we tend to push back!

For instance, when I was playing as a semi-professional athlete, moving around Australia to play with these different teams, I'd get a job quite easily because that would be part of my contract. But then, all of a sudden, that job would finish abruptly, or something didn't work out, or the boss had other plans. There was contrast coming into my existence, and it pushed me on to another experience, and another experience after that. I just kept moving going from job to job to job. At the time, I was thinking, "Oh my, this isn't great for my resume! I'm onto my ninth or tenth job in a matter of three or four years. This is not looking good."

What I realized, however, years later as I founded my company Engage & Grow Global (which is in 80 countries with more than 300 licensed business coaches currently), is that the contrast funneled me in the right direction. It was an amazing gift for me, because I can now talk to people on the factory floor, hospital wards, mining sites, to pubs and clubs, just as easily as I speak to people in the office, in the corporate world, and in government — because I've actually moved through all those areas in some capacity as an employee. At the time, the contrast felt like a hardship and made it difficult for me to find the next job, but I was always actually in perfect play, because I was meant to go there for a certain experience then move to the next and the next.

Contrast occurs when you've got more room for growth to experience, express, and accumulate more information for your life's journey. It will all be good at the end of the day, as long as you keep your vibrations high. Because life is meant to be good, and life is meant to be easy! The person that said 'life was never meant to be easy,' simply had a limiting belief. Your Master mind is always pushing you towards the path of least resistance. When you're off the path, then you're going to get pushed onto a new, happier path. But you've still got to make the choices to move toward your dreams, because the universal law is free will. You get to create what you want. Your intuition will always guide you to the top of the mountain, but many people get themselves off track and end up stumbling down the side of the mountain instead. Enter CONTRAST!

If you're not listening to your Master mind, then you're listening to your Child's mind and that twelve-year-old mentality is probably insisting, "No, no, I don't care. I'm going to go in this direction." If it's not the right direction for your body, mind and soul, you're going to get contrast that will guide you back toward the path that leads to your highest excitement. Sporting injuries are a form of contrast, meaning there's room and opportunity for growth.

You could say contrast is a guiding hand on your shoulder, like a friend guiding you in the right direction. Contrast isn't your enemy– rather it is your friend and mentor, but because we live in this world where your Child's mind is a 12-year-old control freak, people don't always see contrast for the kindness or gift that it is. The Child's mind doesn't always see anything at all, closing its eyes and throwing a tantrum that demands life to change immediately and give it what it wants. That is why a lot of people don't know where they want to go in life. They are literally walking blindfolded through life, and then when they don't get what they want, they blame society or the government, anyone and everyone but themselves. Contrast isn't a slap in the face, which most people see it as. It's purely a guidance system. If you're not where you want to be, that just means you have the opportunity to make more choices and change your world. Contrast is what illuminates those opportunities.

The power of contrast must be managed carefully because it can easily gain momentum if you're not aware. The winds of change are a natural part of life, but the key is to ensure the wind doesn't blow you right off course and into the ravine. All of us have been engulfed in a contrast cyclone, but it's about navigating through it and not allowing the momentum to set in. Don't get caught in the storm! This is where the app comes in.

Abundance

In first world countries, almost everyone is chasing a dollar. Money is the be all and end all, and people lose sight of the fact that abundance comes in many forms. Money is almost always the measuring stick of one's success these days. You have to be careful here though, because by focussing solely on money or material objects as the end game, you are minimising, diminishing or eliminating other precious forms of abundance that are available to help you along the way.

When you are only focussed on money, or when you are fixated on a specific path to a specific type of abundance, you are missing out on all other elements of abundance, and that will slow you down on your road to success. First, releasing control of how and when it comes is of critical importance to receiving abundance. Also, you need to have less of a focus of the form in which it may arrive. Abundance could come to you in the form of synchronicity, as an unexpected inheritance, material gifts, meeting the right person at the right time, expanding your horizons, winning a competition or even winning the lottery! Keep your mind open when you are dreaming of your future successes, and it will flow to you more quickly than ever before.

See It, Feel It, Become It. Close the Gap

That which you feel yourself to be, you are.

If you want to have something new manifest into your life, something powerful, whatever it might be, you must first be able to imagine it. Your imagination is able to do all that you ask in proportion to the degree of your attention. So what kind of attention do you place on your dreams?

In one of Einstein's most famous observations, he said, "Imagination is more important than knowledge. Knowledge is limited. Imagination encircles the world."

Logic will get you from A to B, but imagination will take you everywhere. Make your future dream a present fact by assuming the feeling of the dream fulfilled, and the feeling that would be yours if you were already in possession of your dream. For example, if you want to be All-Australian or All-American, use your imagination to visualize and feel how that actually feels, then hold on to that feeling and practice that feeling until you *become* that feeling every day. When you advance confidently in the direction of your own dreams, and endeavour to live the life which you have imagined, you will meet with success. It will happen, as long as you've done the cleaning down to remove those limiting beliefs that may have been swept under the carpet. The strongest belief will always prevail.

You are where you are today based upon what you believe, and it's not just what you think you believe on the surface. It's also your limiting beliefs that often run deeper that are holding you back from moving into the life you deserve. If you're telling yourself you're not good enough, you're not worthy enough, you're not quick enough, you're not enough, then you end up acting out of that belief system. Quite simply, if you think you can't, you won't. You can't talk defeat and expect to have victory. You can't talk lack, not enough, can't afford it, never get ahead, and expect to have abundance. If your words are poor, you're going to have a poor life.

So often we don't become what we want, because so much of wanting is about living in the space of what we don't have.

That's why Jim Carrey's story is so powerful. He started to act as though he already had it. He would go up to Mulholland Drive. He would drive away saying, thinking, "I already have those things. I just haven't accessed them yet. I believe those things are going to come to me and I'm going to act like they are, so I'm going to move forward in my life in order to draw that to myself in such a way that my actions are in alignment with what I say — I believe."

You can talk yourself out of your dreams. Negative words can keep you from becoming who you were created to be. Don't fall into that trap. Quit calling in defeat. Quit talking about how it's not going to happen. Get focussed, you only have one life in this body. Write down what you want to see happen in life from this very moment forward. Any areas that you're struggling in where you need to improve, write it down like it's already done, and then everyday revisit it. Read It, Feel It, Act It every morning. It's not enough to just think it, you MUST FEEL IT IN YOUR HEART and become that person in your mind's eye. Something happens when we feel it in our heart. This will not only change your outlook; it will change your entire life. It all starts with a choice of thought. Your thoughts become your reality.

Activity #8: Designing the New You (Part 2 of Activity 3)

Again as we did for the first activity for this exercise, we're starting with visualizing your goals in Wealth, Career/Business and Community. We've put together a series of questions for you to answer. Simply take some time to go through the questions and answer them by finding images of what you are working toward in life on the Internet.

Wealth

- Describe what wealthy means to you
- How much money do you earn?
- How much money do you have in the bank?
- What sort of investments do you have?
- What is your net worth?
- What does financial freedom mean to you?

Career/Business

- What do you enjoy doing?
- What are you really good at?
- What sort of work hours do you work?
- Where do you work.... in an office, outside, mobile business?
- What is most rewarding about your work?
- What is your title?
- Who do you work with?

Community

- How can you pay it forward?
- Who do you know that you can help?
- How can you help?
- What causes speak to your soul?
- What local charities can you donate time or money to?
- How can you improve the planet?

Save these photos to your Journal in the Quality Mind app, so they're always at your fingertips for a quick boost to remind you of your dreams. You should also save the images into their own folder on your computer.

Case Study: Trent Dumont

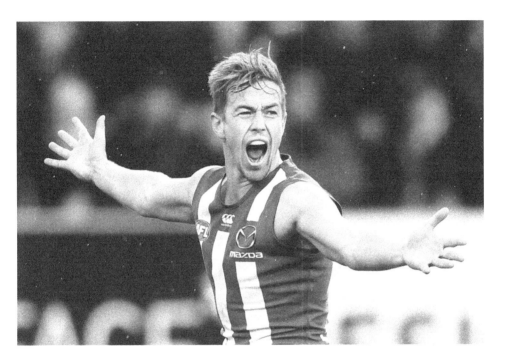

Trent Dumont, North Melbourne FC — AFL Courtesy AFL Photos

Trent Dumont has always had a love for football, and growing up in South Australia, he says that playing football was all he ever did, aside from going to school of course. His parents really pushed education, so footy and school were his focus, and he really excelled in both areas. Trent was recruited by North Melbourne FC (AFL) in 2013 at the age of 18.

"I never experienced any real adversity until I was 19, when I had my first year in the professional sporting industry. It was at the end of the year, sport was going really well, university was going well, I continued my studies, but after the football season finished, in the off-season, I got in an altercation with a taxi driver and I was wrongly accused of robbing him."

"Over two and a half years, I went through the courts and ultimately, two and a half years later, it was found that he was lying, through video footage.

In the meantime though, my name was dragged through the mud, and that lead to some really low points. That's when I started to delve into the mental health space — to try to figure out why I was feeling so miserable. I did some work with professionals around my sporting club in the traditional psychology space. I did a year of that, and then a very respected teammate of mine, Shaun Higgins had a chat to me about Richard. I was really enjoying the work that I was doing, but he said, "If you want to come have a look what Richard does, I feel like you can go to the next level with this sort of stuff. Come to this information session."

"Shaun knew I was interested in the mental health space and the mental side of the game, so he offered the Quality Mind info session to me. I went in with a few teammates, listened to Richard, and to be honest, at first, I thought, "What is this bloke talking about?" But his energy levels are just through the roof, and the more you talk to him the more you realize how simple life can be. He was captivating on so many levels. I knew this bloke meant business and I really liked that about him. He has a bit of an aura about him in terms of his energy levels and how certain he is of himself, and that was a bit captivating and a bit intriguing for me. So that's how I got involved with Quality Mind at the start of this year, before the season started. That's when I started my journey."

"Funnily enough, up until the taxi driver incident, I hadn't experienced any real injuries. But in 2017, when it actually ended in January, I started to really pull up sore, and 2017 was probably the hardest football year of my career in terms of my body. I was going to get MRIs... they knew me by name at the medical centre. I'd walk in, they'd go, "What are you in for this week?" I never really had anything too significant, but it was consistency of little niggles and I just couldn't get rid of them. It was a bit of a learning curve for me."

"Now that I'm seeing Richard, he's given me some great strategies to get rid of the mental blocks, instead of just a bit of guess work in the past. I now know how to always clean down mentally, and I know I'm going to get out there on the field and everything's going to be okay and I'll play the best I can."

"With QM the most important part is the tools. In terms of unlocking that peak energy that you need to perform at the top level, and at the level that you dreamed about, dominating games and what not, that's something that Richard has been able to give me. And it's something that I'm still working on. I definitely haven't nailed it."

"I'm now more aware than ever with how I am thinking and feeling leading up to game days. And if I'm all tied up mentally, as I'm an overthinker sometimes, I can get myself injured. It's amazing how it all lines up when you have the awareness. Now, I'm more aware of everything, and the best part is I know how to handle it. It's just about getting things in place and building it all into your routine, which is why the QM app is so powerful. I will work with Richard for a long time now. The guy that got me into this program, Shaun Higgins, has worked with Richard for five years. He said he was a terrible student early on, but now he's reaping the rewards; he's one of the best players in our competition. I've been working with Richard for about six months now. It's still early days."

"Also, in regards to the program and taking control of your destiny, I like the three-strike policy with the app because that really means you have to commit to yourself and to improving."

"The gameday stuff also appealed to me, because he obviously works closely with athletes. But reflecting on my best games as a player before being in Quality Mind, Richard talks about this 'No-Thing'... you're there, you're performing via your memory and innate which is doing it for you. You're not getting in your own way, you're performing all these skills, and it just feels effortless. You're running fast, but you're not getting tired. When you come off the field after a really good game, you're like, "How did I even do that?" Him talking about being able to tap into that sort of energy level, that was intriguing to me."

"Really, QM just simplifies everything, and I love this quote from Richard: 'Everything is neutral until you give it meaning,' I don't know why sometimes, in your head, you just make these things up and you get caught up."

"It's been a challenging season for our team, too, because we haven't really gone that well, but I've still been able to give pretty rock-solid performances. Going forward, I want to keep being able to work on that and be able to tap into that a bit better. We had our coach sacked half way through this year, so we were in a bit of turmoil. I've been thrown around as a Mr. Fixit a little bit to try and help out the team, but my performance in terms of stats has still increased. I've had more big games than I did last year, so my performance has definitely increased, and I came equal third in the 2019 club championship award — my best performance so far. Even still, I feel like I'm just scratching the surface a bit with this work. I can see the benefits, but where I've been seeing the benefits mostly is just in day-to-day life, energy levels and stuff like that, so now I'm continuously working on the routine of getting that into game day."

"Now that I know I can create the person I want to be, there's no limit on how far I can go. I've done a lot of work with it so far but, also, it's only been six months and I feel like, what are the benefits, or what are the results going to be in five years' time when I've been consistently putting down these solid strategies. What sort of Trent am I going to be in five years' time when I've worked so hard at this mental space, and hopefully I've created the dream that I'm thinking of right now?"

"The creation part of it's probably the key, because I'm not where I want to be in life yet. I've got aspirations to be one of the best players or the best player in the league. And I'd also like to be an inspiration for others: for kids that want to play football, and also to inspire others to look after their mental health and try and be the best person they can be. I want to spread that message."

Do you think that Quality Mind offers an easier and more powerful approach than mainstream sports psychology?

"For sure. The unique teachings, tools and app stands it apart a long way. The app is a big one for me because everyone's got their phone on them, and to have a permanent performance coach in the palm of your hand, I think that's excellent. I can't speak highly enough about the app and the program."

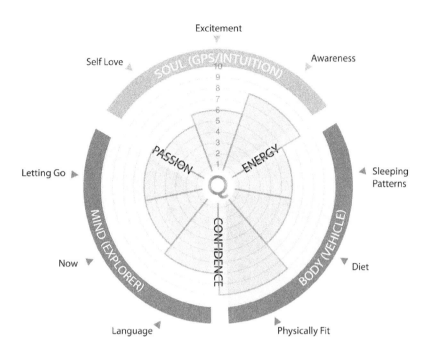

Figure 1: Trent Dumont when perfoming inconsistently.

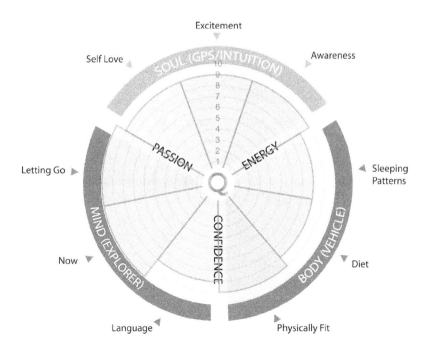

Figure 2: Trent Dumont when performing consistently.

Case Study: Laura Attard

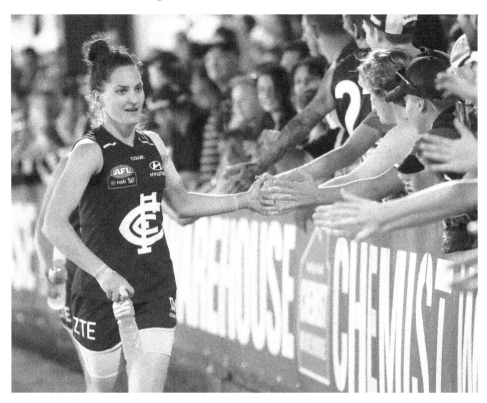

Laura Attard with Carlton FC, AFL — Courtesy AFL Photos

Laura Attard came from a sporting family. Her brothers were both heavily involved in sport, and her sister in dance. Laura always loved footy, and when she was eight years old, she started going to local Auskick with her brother. Auskick is like the junior version of AFL, and it was there that she developed a strong passion for the game.

"At the age of 12 I was told I couldn't play the junior level of football because it was only for boys. So then I started playing netball and doing squad swimming. I used to go and watch my brothers play football all the time, and my dad coaching them. I longed to play. Then at 18 a women's football league was being formed, and that's when I saw my chance and I started playing footy at a senior level."

"After three years I decided that I wanted to challenge myself, and I went to the Premier Division. During that period I always tried out for state squads and country metro squads and representative programs, but I would find that I'd get through the first few cuts, but I wouldn't quite make the final cut. Or if I was having a particularly good year that year, something always happened where I'd get injured and I wouldn't actually play on to get picked."

"There are a couple of times I did get selected but had to withdraw because I'd break my arm or I'd ruptured my medial ligament in my knee and things like that. That was sort of the trend of my footy career. I loved it more than anything, but I just never really made it to the highest level."

"Then in 2015 the AFL announced that they were going to bring in the AFLW competition, which was a national football competition. I was super excited to say the least, and I made a decision that this has to be it for me. I had to make this competition. It just so happened at the time I was at work teaching and I was reading the Herald Sun newspaper on my lunch break. I saw an article in the back of the sports section about Shaun Higgins and Easton Wood raving on about Quality Mind."

"The article really spoke to me. It was one of those funny things to come across because when I read it I thought 'that's been my career'. Both Shaun and Easton had struggled with injury and consistency at the top level. I just thought, you know, for me, one of the biggest things holding me back was the fact that I kept getting injured. Second, there was the fact that I probably just didn't believe in myself enough. It got me excited about jumping in and seeing what kind of difference it would have on me as I had nothing to lose. So I jumped on the internet, googled Richard and sent him an email."

Enter Richard

"Richard was really energetic, he was very passionate, and he said lets chat, so that's what we did. My first impressions were that he was really honest with his expectations — if I was going to get involved then I must be 110% serious, and I had to fully commit, or he would not work with me."

"I went home and I was probably a little bit sceptical as it wasn't a traditional approach. If I had gone to another sports psychologist they would ask me to pay a consulting fee and come back when I'm ready."

"So I went home and chatted to my partner about it and said, you know, this is something that I really want and I feel like I need to give it a go. So I decided to commit to the program, and within three or four weeks I knew that it was definitely the right decision."

"Funnily enough around this time, my family and friends started making comments that I seemed, you know, a little bit lighter, a little bit happier, all those sorts of things. And the only person that knew I was doing the program was my partner, so they just thought my happiness was because of my partner. They're like 'Tiarna's having a really great impact on you' and I'm like, yeah, yeah, she is, isn't she? So that was quite funny!"

Injured, Tired & Torn

"Since starting the program in 2015 I have not missed a game through injury, and I really have played the most consistent football of my career. In the past I had season ending injuries such as a complete rupture of my medial ligament in my knee, which had me in a full leg brace for 12 weeks. I broke my arm at one point and ended with a plate and seven screws in it. That had me out of the game for 12 weeks. I had done an AC injury of my left shoulder that had me in a sling for eight weeks. I had some pretty serious injuries that kept me out of the game and required operations, etc."

"Whereas, since starting Quality Mind, nothing at all has kept me off the track. The work is on my mind and yet the impact on my body has been so positive."

"A big part of the program that impacted me, among so many other things, is what Richard teaches around dissolving limiting beliefs. There is an easy way to uncover these by being honest with yourself about your belief systems of what you're capable of. That has been probably the most valuable thing. Even just things like the way that people perceived me as a person. That was a limiting belief of my own and in a sense was holding me back from my own relationships with people. It became a program that was a lot more than just my sporting career, it impacted every facet of my life."

Future

"I think the future is really exciting. I feel like there's unlimited possibilities now. Prior to Quality Mind, I probably felt like I had limited avenues that I could follow in life. Whereas, now it's kind of like whatever I'm excited about I feel like I can follow. I find that there's always doors opening in whatever I'm doing. I just get excited about that process, as well. I no longer feel anxious when a new opportunity presents, or worry about failing. I just think, 'well let's go and jump in and follow and see where it goes.' It's pretty exciting really!"

"Quality Mind can work for anyone — regardless of which sport they might engage in. There's a multifaceted approach and it's for people in business, it's for people in sport, it's for people in their everyday lives. As I said, it's impacted me in every aspect of my life."

"I would absolutely recommend the program, and it was great fun working with Richard. We definitely challenged each other at times, which is probably what's required to really get something out of it. He's a super-energetic person, he's really passionate about what he does and it was really enjoyable to work one-on-one with him."

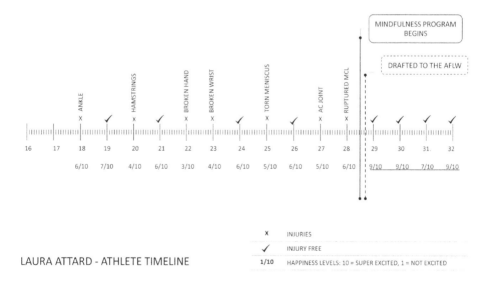

Laura Attard, General Life & Sport Timeline

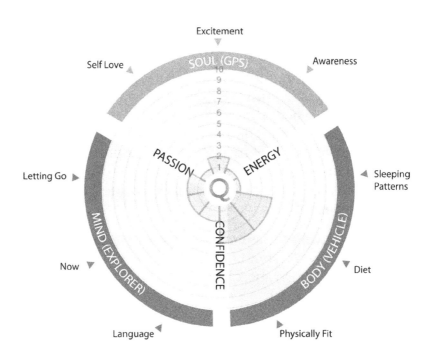

Figure 1: Laura Attard — Before her QM Journey Begun

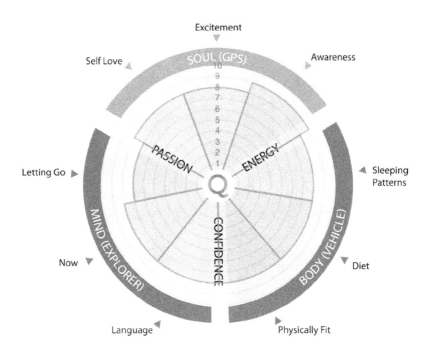

Figure 2: Laura Attard — Today and during her Quality Mind Journey

Step #5: Live
QM Performance Plan

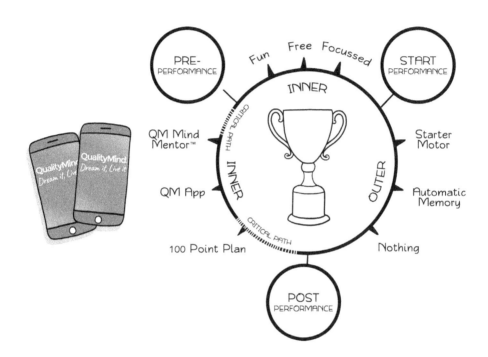

Quality Mind — Elite Athlete Performance Plan

As an elite athlete, your success is predominantly determined by your off-field performance. In fact, 70% of your on-field performance is determined in the lead up to, and after the performance. Throughout the years of training in your sporting profession, your memory (or hard drive) has been collecting data that is then stored away, ready to access at a later date. However, much like a computer, if you don't upgrade your system and clean out your folders regularly, things will slow down and your performance will be tainted. This is more important today than ever before, because of the added pressures we are bombarded with in modern day life. The Quality Mind performance plan takes this into account. So let me walk you through our proven and powerful performance plan.

Stage One — Pre-Performance:

You arrive at the stadium and the goal is to have fun and feel free, but with a determined focus to dominate. You can feel the energy building in your heart centre, but there is no need to fully switch on until the coach takes centre stage.

Stage Two — Start Performance:

Now you are running out onto the field ready to begin your performance. This is when you bring in your starter motor, and the starter motor's job is to fire the engine to get the vehicle moving. The starter motor is your Master coming through and preparing you with the fuel to fire on all cylinders once the flag is dropped. Your starter motor may be a carefully chosen short power statement that is all consuming and will impact your entire being via the vibration of the words. For example:

- It's my time to shine
- Get the %$#@ out of my way
- It's time to dominate
- I am All-Australian / All-American
- This is my stage
- This game is mine to own
- I am a true leader

Now that you're in the game and you have become part of the game, it's time to open up your hard drive to allow your automatic memory through. You're now at a stage where you are playing on instinct and memory, and you're not consciously investing too much energy in thinking through the play.

Now you're in the zone, which is the holy grail of performance. Here, you are dancing through the performance and everything seems easy and seamless. Here, the game is flowing to you as though you are the creator of the game, as opposed to everyone else who is chasing the game and feeling exhausted. Your energy levels are supreme, and nothing seems to phase you. You are in flow.

Athletes know when they've been in this space because it's hard to remember the performance. This is because your automatic memory has taken over and you are not consciously all there.

Stage Three — Post Performance:

This is the critical path. The 70%.

Myself or one of our Mind Mentors will personally walk you through this critical process, should you join our program!

We are also always seeking to add Mind Mentors to our global team, should this be of interest.

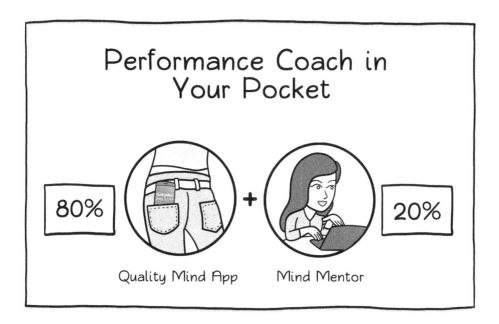

To Truly Live — Live With Heart

To Truly Live — we must live with Heart, again, it's all in the science! New studies are showing that the human heart is the strongest biological generator of electrical fields and magnetic fields in the human body. So our heart has the ability to generate the very fields that our world is made up of. And our own physics textbooks say if you want to change your reality, you have to change either the electrical fields or magnetic fields around you.

Science tells us that when we have a feeling in our heart, we are actually creating the electrical and magnetic waves that change the quality of the atoms of our world. They literally interrupt the flow of space and time and rearrange the stuff this world is made of. So the heart it seems, truly is our MOST powerful creator AND it literally has the means to manifest our reality!

The bottom line to all of this, and this is what the ancient traditions have always said, is that we're invited to feel the feelings inside our heart for the things that we would like to experience in our lives. To feel as if they've already happened, rather than asking for them to happen and feeling powerless in our world, which we all do from time to time.

It sounds like hocus pocus, until we understand that when we have that feeling we're creating the electrical and the magnetic template. It's the blueprint in our heart that the quantum stuff of our universe congeals around to give us the reality that matches what it is that we've felt.

The heart is about 100 times stronger electrically than the human brain. And the heart is about 5,000 times stronger magnetically than the human brain. So if we're going to create an electrical or a magnetic field that affects our reality, it can't be done with thought alone. It's much easier to feel with our hearts.

We model and we simulate with our brain, so our brain creates the image of what it is we like to see and what it is we like to experience. And once we have that locked into place, we can feel the feeling of gratitude and appreciation for what has already happened, and give power to what it is that we're thinking. And this is a very powerful internal technology that apparently was lost to the West about two centuries ago. And the instructions are just now being found in many of the texts that have been recovered in the last 100 years.

So the feeling is what actually creates, and if the feeling is what creates, then you've got to give that field something to work with so it can show you what it is that you're creating. Why not feel what it is that you'd like to experience so the field can give that back to you, rather than feeling the things that you don't have or you don't want, because that gets back to you as well.

So it's this little subtle shift into thinking from the outcome rather than thinking from a place of lack and hoping something changes. And the feeling that we're creating is very closely associated with what we call belief. Belief and feeling both occur in the heart, and when you have a belief about something, you've usually got really strong feelings about that belief.

So truly believe it, and you will achieve it. How good is that!

7 Non Negotiables

A reasonable sports career can be achieved by anyone with the talent who is already in the industry, but if you want a great sports career, you must commit to leading a great life, to doing things the majority do not do, and to thinking like the minority, not like the majority.

Here are seven principles to live by for an abundant, happy, successful sporting career and life.

Non Negotiable #1: the first principle to live by is that one day you will be gone. It may be in 50 years, it may be in 50 weeks. It may be next week or even today. I don't know. You don't know. Nobody knows, and rather than live in fear of this, we should embrace the fact that this life is short, precious and unpredictable. And in knowing this, we must live fully for today. It is not a recipe for recklessness, but rather a recipe to give your all today, to give your very best today in everything you do, to give your greatest energy to this day, to your family, to everyone you encounter today.

It is a reminder for you to be your best self in each moment. What if you were gone tomorrow? What would they speak of you? What can you do that will leave a lasting positive memory in the lives of everyone you come into contact with? It's about being light-hearted, and knowing that in the end, none of this stuff matters. The only thing that ever matters is how happy you were with your time here on planet earth. Did you achieve what you wanted to achieve? Did you make others feel loved? It is about knowing that things can never go with you in the end, and remembering that we are going to die is the greatest reminder we can have in our daily lives because it keeps us focused on what's really important and what is real.

Non-Negotiable #2: there is nothing you cannot be, do or have. Period! If there has been someone, even one person on this planet that has done it before, that means you can too. It doesn't mean it will be easy, but it does mean it's possible, and as long as it is possible, you can work towards it. You can make a plan. Learn what needs to be done for you to live your craziest, most abundant life — a life most would consider impossible. But you know, impossible, broken down, states I am possible. You know impossible broken down is simply the process of making a plan and being willing to work for that plan.

Non-Negotiable #3: always charge towards your highest excitement. Ask yourself this question about everything you do in your life. Does this make me happy? If the answer is no, ask yourself will this sacrifice I am making lead to more happiness in the long term? If not, you should let it go.

Non-Negotiable #4: be yourself. Always. No exceptions. It's such a tragedy to see so many people on this planet living lives they don't want to live just because they listened to other people who did the same. The only way you can live happy in this life, the only way you can be successful, is if you be you. Learn about yourself — Know Thyself, Accept Thyself, Become The Conscious Creator moment by moment.

Non-Negotiable #5: everything you need is already within you. In this world, we see endless examples of people who seemingly have it all, materially speaking, but they are empty inside.

A beggar had been sitting on the side of the road for over thirty years. One day a stranger walked by. "Spare some change?" mumbled the beggar, mechanically holding out his old baseball cap. "I have nothing to give you," said the stranger! Then he asked "what's that you're sitting on?" "Nothing," replied the beggar, "just an old box. I've been sitting on it for as long as I can remember." "Ever looked inside?" asked the stranger. "No," said the beggar. "What's the point, there is nothing in there." "Have a look inside," insisted the stranger. The beggar managed to ply open the lid, and with astonishment, disbelief and elation, he saw that the box was filled with gold.

This parable lays out the very essence of human suffering. We are always looking externally for answers to our problems, for validation, for security, for love, but everything you ever need can be found within.

The solution is found in our minds and in our hearts. Because our thoughts are the cause of all suffering.

Non-Negotiable #6: the most important moment in everyday is the first moment when you wake up in the morning. Take full control of your state as soon as you register back into this reality. The reason why is chemical. Cortisol is nature's built-in alarm system. It's your body's main stress hormone. It works with certain parts of your brain to control your mood, motivation and fear. It's best known for helping fuel your body's "fight-or-flight" instinct in a crisis, and when we wake up a lot of the time we fly off into worry about the day ahead or the day that was.

This must stop! If you wake stressed, then don't allow momentum to kick in. Pick up your QM app, select one of the walking meditations and hit the beat, or stay there in bed and select a high vibration meditation that will get you focussed on living in your future self. Help yourself dream with clarity — See it, Feel it, and Become it. Stay in that state for as long as possible.

Non-Negotiable #7: whatever you focus on and desire with all your heart, you can create. If you search for negativity in this world, you will find plenty of it. If you search for hate, anger, violence, and sadness, you will find it, but the same is true on the flip side. If your only intention is to search for the good, you will find only the good, and whatever meaning you give your life becomes your life. We choose our own reality by the meaning we give each moment in our lives. Make it your intention to look for the good in your life, to notice the good in others, to be grateful for what you do have, to see challenges as opportunities to show your true character.

Remember: what you give your attention to will become your experience in life. Practice seeing the good in your life and in others. Think the best, expect the best, and always ask yourself, how can this benefit my life? Leave who you were behind and create the next and best version of yourself. Love who you are, get excited, and look forward to who you are becoming!

Backmatter

Acknowledgments

- HeartMath.com graphics and information courtesy of HeartMath Institute
- AFL Images of athletes Courtesy AFL Photos
- **Herald Sun** — www.qualitymindglobal.com/blog/article/easton-wood-shaun-higgins-credit-injury-free-mind-coach-with-career-best-seasons
- **Kitmanlabs** — www.kitmanlabs.com/what-is-the-real-cost-of-injuries-in-professional-sport/

Disclaimer:

This book details the author's personal experiences with and opinions about *mindfulness and managing stress*. The author is not a registered healthcare provider.

The author and publisher are providing this book and its contents on an "as is" basis and make no representations or warranties of any kind with respect to this book or its contents. The author and publisher disclaim all such representations and warranties, including for example warranties of merchantability and healthcare for a particular purpose. In addition, the publisher does not represent or warrant that the information accessible via this book is accurate, complete or current.

The statements made about products and services have not been evaluated by the *Australian* or U.S. Food and Drug Administration. They are not intended to diagnose, treat, cure, or prevent any condition or disease. Please consult with your own physician or healthcare specialist regarding the suggestions and recommendations made in this book.

Except as specifically stated in this book, neither the author or publisher, nor any authors, contributors, or other representatives will be liable for damages arising out of or in connection with the use of this book.

This is a comprehensive limitation of liability that applies to all damages of any kind, including (without limitation) compensatory; direct, indirect or consequential damages; loss of data, income or profit; loss of or damage to property and claims of third parties.

You understand that this book is not intended as a substitute for consultation with a licensed healthcare practitioner, such as your physician. Before you begin any healthcare program, or change your lifestyle in any way, you will consult your physician or another licensed healthcare practitioner to ensure that you are in good health and that the examples contained in this book will not harm you.

This book provides content related to physical and/or mental health issues. As such, use of this book implies your acceptance of this disclaimer.

About the Author

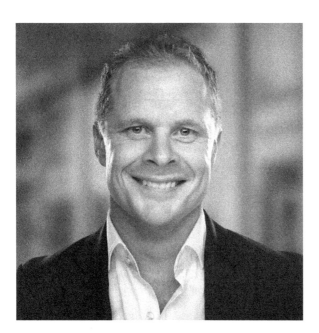

Richard Maloney is the founder and Director of Engage & Grow Global and founder and CEO of Quality Mind Global. With over 20 years of experience in the sports industry, and having worked with hundreds of elite athletes, Rich has proven time and time again that the body is led by the mind. Now, he has a unique and tangible system designed to minimize or eliminate injuries from athletes through systematic mental training, allowing you to unlock your ultimate sports capability and your true potential, in both sport and in life.

It all started for Richard, when at the age of 18, he was recruited to play for his beloved, St Kilda Football Club (AFL). This was the epitome of success for a footballer, playing at the most elite level in Australia. It seemed like a dream come true, and yet, what he gained there was a very stark and unnerving realization that he wasn't mentally equipped to handle the immense pressure that came with being an elite sportsman. Richard was already battling demons in his personal life, and the stress proved all too much. He chose to walk away from his lifelong dream, but this failure stayed with him, and it ultimately drove him to build his 'Quality Mind' business.

Now 44 years old, Richard has been associated with six elite Australian sports organisations, including the Western Bulldogs Football Club (AFL) as their Leadership and Culture Coach. He has helped 32 local sporting teams win premierships, and he has brought over 50 teams to finals. Richard is also the founder, creator and owner of two incredibly successful businesses;

Engage & Grow Global, which is making a huge global impact on employee happiness in the workplace. With over 300 Employee Engagement licensees now running Richards' systems in 35 countries, they bring the colour back in to people's lives and workplaces.

And Quality Mind Global, which has over 200 clients in 15 countries, as well as Quality Mind Mentor Licensees in 7 countries.

With the development of Quality Mind, what started as a way of simply removing injuries in elite athletes by unlocking their minds, has now opened the door for every person to release the magic of mental transformation into their lives. Richard's homegrown system, the Maloney Method, has been integrated into a unique, proven, step by step system that has helped hundreds of people remove the obstacles holding them back from living the life of their dreams. Now, with the recent introduction of the game changing Quality Mind app, he is literally changing lives every day.

Richard has been a headline speaker at many industry conferences and events, and he has spoken in 15 countries. He is the author of The Minds of Winning Teams: Creating Team Success Through Engagement & Culture and co-author, alongside Dr. Marshall Goldsmith, Brad Sugars and Mark Thompson of Engage & Grow: 6 Steps to Building Highly Engaged Employees.

Richard was also recognized as a finalist in the 2016, 2017 & 2018 Australian Optus Business Awards as Business Leader of the Year and Export Business of the Year and as a finalist for the 2017 Telstra Victorian Micro Business of the Year.

Richard lives in Melbourne, Australia, with his wife Kristen and their three young daughters.

You can learn more about Quality Mind Global and Engage & Grow Global via these links below.

www.qualitymindglobal.com
www.engageandgrowglobal.com

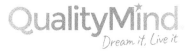

Discover the secret to consistent, injury free, powerful performances.

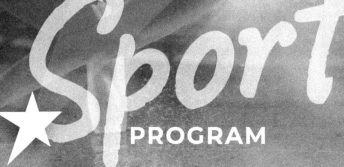

Sport
PROGRAM

qualitymindglobal.com

QualityMind

Are your energy levels and recovery time suffering? Is your mindset limiting your physical progression? Do you wish you could free yourself from the negative thought patterns stopping you from reaching your true potential?

The Quality Mind Sport Program is a five-step approach tailored to your needs by your personal Mind Mentor™. With their support in the Quality Mind app, you'll learn practical mental tools designed to align your mind, body and soul – all so you can reach your true potential.

How & why it works

We use tried-and-tested strategies specifically for athletes

In over two decades, our founder Richard Maloney has helped 32 sporting teams win championships, 100+ athletes and six elite Australian sports organizations conquer their demons. Our program is best-in-class mental development for high-performance athletes.

You have access to personalized mentorship

We give you access to a personal Mind Mentor™, either face to face or online, to help implement our proven mental tools.

You pick the milestones

Whether it's success in sport, beating your personal best or simply improving your overall fitness, you set the targets. We'll create a trackable plan to get you there both mentally and physically.

We offer visible goals and accountability

Our Quality Mind App is designed to map out your masterplan and monitor your progress. That means both your app and your Mind Mentor™ will keep you on track - even on the days when you're not at your best.

There's a maintenance program

Getting your head straight is one thing, but keeping it there requires ongoing effort. We offer a maintenance program that ensures steady physical improvement long after you've completed the more intensive programs.

Behind Quality Mind

At 18, our founder Richard Maloney was unable to overcome his own emotional roadblocks – and it cost him his career in professional football. It was this loss that kick-started his journey cultivating the mental tools to effectively help people push though their fears, thought patterns and emotional ruts.

Quality Mind's model is a blend of:

- Neuroscience
- Positive Psychology
- HeartMath Technology
- Neuro Linguistic Programming (NLP)
- Ancient Philosophies

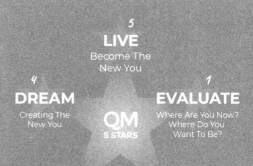

5 LIVE — Become The New You

4 DREAM — Creating The New You

QM 5 STARS

1 EVALUATE — Where Are You Now? Where Do You Want To Be?

3 CLEAN — Making Room For The New

2 RETRAIN — Discovering Another Way

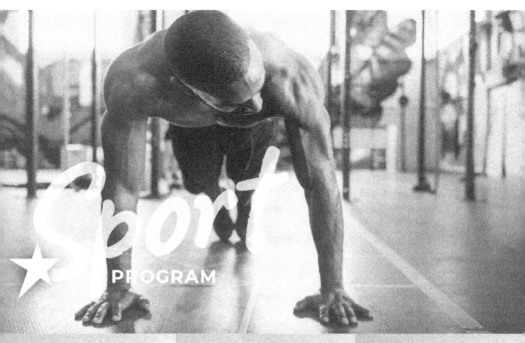

Sport PROGRAM

Junior Athletes

Developing Mental Foundations

Planning to push yourself towards physical improvement is simple. But implementation is another story. Your mind doesn't always back your goals – even if they're as clear as day. This program will help you realign your thoughts and motivations with your current aspirations. (12-16 years)

Aspiring Elite Athletes

Prepare mentally for Elite

When you're trying to reach the next level, pushing your body to new limits, it can be frustrating if your mind isn't pulling its weight. This program will help you identify and remove negative thought patterns or limiting beliefs that are holding you back from upping your game. Helping you design and create your elite sporting dreams. (16+ years)

Elite Athletes

Excelling and Dominating

How do you stay focused, motivated and injury-free under such high levels of pressure in elite sport? You have to use every tool at your disposal – most importantly your mind. Quality Mind is designed to give you the tools you need to manage your stress on a day-to-day basis and align your thoughts with your objectives rather than your anxieties.

Quality Mind is designed to help you:

- Eliminate thoughts that clutter your focus
- Identify and overcome roadblocks limiting performance
- Manage thought patterns to support your goals
- Gain emotional clarity
- Enhance mental energy
- Achieve higher levels of physicality
- Consistently build towards a stronger, healthier body and mind
- Reduce or eliminate risk of injury
- Rest effectively, mind and body
- Fast-track recovery from current injuries
- Remove anxiety
- Manage pressure

qualitymindglobal.com

3 of our most popular packages

Workshops

INTRODUCTION TO MINDFULNESS: Discover the fundamentals of building a Quality Mind, including how to get started and why it can help you.

INJURY FREE: Reduce and eliminate injuries through mental exercises and proven mindfulness techniques. Recover faster and stay fit for longer.

CONSISTENT PERFORMANCE: Deliver your best every time you step out onto the field. Eradicate underlying fears and make first-class performance a habit.

STRESS MANAGEMENT: Learn how best to deal with the pressures of elite sport and high-stress situations. Declutter your mind and find calm in the storm.

LEADERSHIP: Unlock your leadership potential with psychological triggers and confidence tactics. Develop the skills needed to stand up and be counted.

Crews

CONNECT CREW: A 3-6 month program with between 5 and 15 participants. You'll have full access to the Quality Mind App and our Quality Mind community, including bespoke support from your Mind Mentor through the app and on live webinars.

POWER CREW: A month-by-month program with up to 100 participants. Weekly sessions will focus on themes around performing to your potential and coping with setbacks.

STAY CONNECTED CREW: A personal, online program designed to support you after you've completed the Connect Crew or the Power Crew. It's the best way to keep yourself on track in building your Quality Mind.

Tailored Programs

Powerful and personal development plans tailored to you. You'll tap into Richard's priceless experience through your Mind Mentor™ with one to one support, as well as gain access to a collection of webinars, workshops and your Quality Mind app.

Dream it, Live it

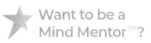 **Want to be a Mind Mentor™?**

Does the happiness and success of others play a bit part in your life? Do you want to stay connected to the sport you love – but aren't sure how?

Here's how you can do exactly that by being a licensed Mind Mentor™. Live and breathe the Quality Mind program for at least three months and you'll be eligible to apply.

Our client reviews

"I needed to come at my issues from a different angle because everything else just wasn't working... After the first month I could see that I was changing and there was a way out of the hole I'd dug for myself. Now I'm playing some of the best footy of my career."
EASTON WOOD, AUSTRALIAN RULES FOOTBALL ATHLETE

"The Quality Mind program has been a complete game changer for my footy. Starting the program back in 2013 when I was injured for the year, the following year I played 22 games out of 22, something I'd never been able to do before. It saved my career!"
SHAUN HIGGINS, AUSTRALIAN RULES FOOTBALL ATHLETE

"I can see colleagues and athletes around me crumbling under the pressure. I can relate, if I hadn't been on this journey and grasped this program, I would definitely be in the situation they are. Quality Mind has changed my life, it is turning my dreams into reality."
DR TIARNA ERNST, OBSTETRICS & GYNAECOLOGY, WOMENS AUSTRALIAN RULES FOOTBALL ATHLETE

qualitymindglobal.com

DOWNLOAD NOW

Simply call
1300 QMLIFE or **1300 765 433**
Email us at
info@qualitymindglobal.com
Find us online
www.qualitymindglobal.com

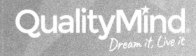

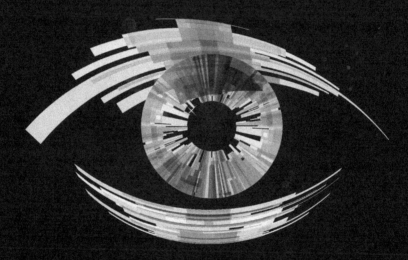

CPSIA information can be obtained
at www.ICGtesting.com
Printed in the USA
BVHW042022281119
565100BV00008B/78/P